Disorderly Movements

"I knew her as Dr. Anne Young, Chair of the Department of Neurology at Harvard Medical School. Now I know her journey from rebel-adolescent to wife/parent and determined physician/researcher. This is an honest memoir of love and loss transformed into a life of deep meaning and legacy. This memoir would be particularly appreciated by anyone already in, or considering a future in, medicine. Yet, as my own personal neurologist, I will always consider her as Dr. Anne Young: the Queen of Neurology – and now I know why I liked her so much not only as a physician, but as a human."

Dr. Jill Bolte Taylor
Author of *My Stroke of Insight and Whole Brain Living*
Time 100 Most Influential

"Dr. Anne Young is a true rock star of neurology and her amazing story is an inspiration for all seeking to overcome life's obstacles to reach the highest pinnacles of success. *Disorderly Movements* is a triumph of human spirit and pure brilliance!!"

Dr. Rudolph E. Tanzi
New York Times Bestselling Author
Joseph P. and Rose F. Kennedy Professor of Neurology,
Harvard University and Massachusetts General Hospital

"When I knew Anne Young years ago at Vassar College, I thought she was wild and interesting and a little crazy. I never thought that girl would evolve into the celebrated and deeply caring neuroscientist she has become. What does one get when one combines scientific brilliance, addiction, ambition, compassion, humor, and devastating loss? Great drama. A dear friend. And Dr. Anne Young's page-turner of a memoir, *Disorderly Movements*."

Rebecca Eaton, Executive Producer Emerita, *MASTERPIECE* on PBS

Disorderly Movements

A Neurologist's Adventures in the Lab and Life

Anne Buckingham Young

Massachusetts General Hospital

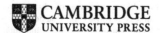
CAMBRIDGE
UNIVERSITY PRESS

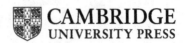

CAMBRIDGE
UNIVERSITY PRESS

Shaftesbury Road, Cambridge CB2 8EA, United Kingdom

One Liberty Plaza, 20th Floor, New York, NY 10006, USA

477 Williamstown Road, Port Melbourne, VIC 3207, Australia

314–321, 3rd Floor, Plot 3, Splendor Forum, Jasola District Centre,
New Delhi – 110025, India

103 Penang Road, #05–06/07, Visioncrest Commercial, Singapore 238467

Cambridge University Press is part of Cambridge University Press & Assessment,
a department of the University of Cambridge.

We share the University's mission to contribute to society through the pursuit of
education, learning and research at the highest international levels of excellence.

www.cambridge.org
Information on this title: www.cambridge.org/9781009492904

DOI: 10.1017/9781009492898

First published 2025

A catalogue record for this publication is available from the British Library

*A Cataloging-in-Publication data record for this book is available from the Library of
Congress*

ISBN 978-1-009-49290-4 Paperback

To Jack and Nancy and my daughters, Jessie and Ellen

Contents

Contents

Foreword

The first time I heard of Anne Young was when a lab friend told me she was about to be eaten alive. I was doing my MD–PhD thesis on motor control, and he and I both knew her work because she had revolutionized our field. Until then, to me she had only been a name at the top of important research papers. My friend told me that Anne was a brilliant scientist and clinician who had just come to Boston as the neurology chair of Massachusetts General Hospital (MGH), an institution that we Bostonians believed to be Man's Greatest Hospital. He said Anne was the only woman ever to chair an MGH department and was very young to be a chair because she had done an MD–PhD in only five years – a joint degree that we both knew firsthand took most trainees many years longer. The MGH neurology department had long been organized into fiefdoms – units such as stroke and epilepsy – and the elderly unit directors would surely defend their territory and squash her.

Because I hoped to do a neurology residency at MGH, Anne Young's fate mattered to me. I tried to reassure myself that, if she had managed to escape the grip of her graduation committee in only five years, she would have strategies for dealing with MGH's hierarchy too. Anne would no doubt attend the upcoming annual Society for Neuroscience convention, and we would probably go to the same movement control poster sessions. It would be fun to shadow her and check out what she was like. My friend told me it would be easy to spot her in the conference crowds by her unusual ex-hippy hairdo, a long ponytail tied over her right ear.

During the convention, my spying added an extra level of amusement to the heady buzz of 10,000 neuroscientists exchanging ideas at top speed. Anne moved from poster to poster; I followed. She didn't seem to be the wispy creature my friend's words had made me fear. I decided her jeans and scruffy backpack, so much less formal than most MDs, showed her independence. She radiated good humor and generosity, stopping even at the sad little student posters most lab heads passed by. Her questions to other scientists were penetrating, but also friendly invitations to explore a subject more deeply.

I tried to take mental notes on how she managed to be both pugnacious and disarming. She often introduced herself to poster presenters by saying "I can't read. Can you summarize your poster for me?" Years later, she told me she wasn't just playing dumb – she has mild dyslexia. She would get her husband Jack to read the scientific papers they needed for their research, and then she and he would discuss them. In our publish-or-perish profession, it is better to be a producer than a consumer. Perhaps her discomfort with scientific prose helps her be such an engaging communicator.

A few days later in the same conference, I went to a session of short talks that Anne moderated. To keep long-winded speakers from going overtime, talk session moderators often rely on loud buzzers or abrupt interruptions. Anne's approach was different. As the time limit approached, she would stand up silently and sidle nearer and nearer to the lecturer. Most speakers quickly finished their talk, and audiences loved her pantomime. Only a few orators were so deeply self-absorbed that they didn't sense her coming toward them with her invisible vaudeville hook. Even they eventually heard the crowd's roars of laughter and, almost on time, would shut up.

Two years after that meeting, I went to my MGH internship interview, a ritual infamous among applicants for having a faculty-to-student ratio of five to one. I sat in front of the line of five dark suits, and wondered if I should regret not having bothered to buy the blue blazer I had seen all the other applicants wearing. "Why do you want to come to this august institution?" asked one of the dark suits in a half-ironic, half-pompous tone. "Because I'm an Anne Young wannabe," I replied, flipping my long ponytail to hang by my right ear. They liked my answer; Anne was already well respected at MGH. She had somehow defanged her unit chiefs' power, putting each unit's revenues into a fund that she controlled, yet she had mysteriously managed to win their loyalty at the same time.

During my MGH training, I studied both neurology and Anne. How did she do so much, and get away with it? She was brilliant, of course, but that was commonplace at Harvard. She had amazing social skills, despite professing to be a shy introvert. If she had taught herself to act like that, could the rest of us?

Trainees like me, who struggled to control our temper, marveled at how Anne got away with expressing anger. She was famously explosive – although she directed most of her blasts at colleagues and superiors and usually spared us residents.

One of Anne's most public blow-ups came at the end of a neurology grand rounds lecture. The speaker was an unremarkable doctor from another department who had droned on and on, touting a new drug he claimed could treat Alzheimer's disease. Our department held grand rounds in the 200-year-old former surgical theater called the Ether Dome. Residents sat in the cramped nosebleed seats, leaning forward so our head didn't touch the dome, and struggled to stay awake. The seats in that top row were old leather bicycle-style saddles on long iron poles, and we knew that, if we fell asleep, we would fall off our pole with a crash the dome would amplify.

Anne, far below us in the front row, always asked the first question after a talk. Usually, it was an insightful and entertaining query that would help us wake up before going back to ward work. This time, though, she didn't ask a question. She stood up to her full height and chewed the speaker out with great force. She told him he should be ashamed of himself. He blurred fact and fantasy, she said, and couldn't be trusted. The data were slimy with pharma company influence. She finished by announcing: "You! Are! Fired!" with such conviction that it was days before I realized she couldn't really fire him; he was not in her department. Nonetheless, the speaker disappeared like a minor comic book villain in a puff of smoke. He was never heard of again.

The event lived on in institutional memory. The residents re-enacted it in their year's-end skit. Fifteen years later, at Anne's retirement party, one colleague's nostalgic tribute recounted her grand rounds fury and showed a slide of Judith beheading Holofernes.

Did Anne inspire our loyalty and hard work because of, or despite, her occasional rages? One way she kept from alienating people was that she didn't stay angry long and could later discuss the same subject calmly. She usually made it clear that she hated the sin, not the sinner. As a former Mass General colleague once told me cheerfully after a faculty feedback session: "She nailed my head to the wall! But I deserved it."

Women, and many men, often worry their getting angry will open them to others' aggression. When their hesitation makes their anger sound sulky or weak, though, it only encourages counterattack. Anne, in the heat of her anger, was fearless and burned with sincere righteousness. Later, if she found she had been wrong, she would retract her position with such certainty that her apology didn't weaken her, it impressed others with her open-mindedness.

I watched how Anne's bluntness made people admire her as a straight shooter, and how her offhand exposure of her own weak points made her seem so confident that she could afford to be humble. She generously gave us junior staff and trainees explicit career advice at her own expense. For instance, she would tell the senior residents not to let her know they would love to stay on as staff at MGH, because it would just decrease their bargaining power with her. She encouraged them to interview at competing institutions. "You may find a place that is better for you. Even if you don't, at least you'll get job offers you can tell me about. Use their offers to negotiate with me for a salary increase."

To advance my study of Anne, I often ran my theories past her, to see if they matched her own self-perception. They usually didn't. For instance, when I praised her confident uses of anger and self-disclosure, she said forcefully, "No, I am timid! I'm afraid of driving across bridges. I secretly think everyone hates me. My rage attacks are just symptoms of my mood lability." Of course, a symptom can also be a strength when deployed effectively. But how could Anne be confident and relaxed, and yet also ashamed and self-critical? Is it a symptom that she can keep two sides of her character so separate? Or a strength?

Anne was tolerant of staff who didn't follow her plan for them. One time I admitted to her that I was neglecting my research work to write a general-audience book about hypergraphia and writer's block. She said, as she has said to many others, that I should do whatever I wanted, as long as it was interesting. After my book was published and she read it, she told me it had motivated her to write a book herself, a memoir. She soon came back with a manuscript so much livelier and more disinhibited than the ponderous memoirs of her emeritus colleagues that her long-time executive secretary told her "You can't publish that until after you retire, or you'll get fired!" Anne, always open to learning from others, took her advice.

Anne is a great oral storyteller. Her residents and junior staff loved when she switched from her efficient doctor voice to her rich, yarn-spinning cadence. She told us about taking the Medical College Admission Test with a hangover from attending a Kentucky Derby party the night before. When I was pregnant, she told me not to be an over-anxious parent the way she had been: she had measured her children's head circumference every day for their first year, so she could check if they were developing a brain tumor. Her research tales included the time when she and her best friend and collaborator Nancy Wexler, during their yearly boat trip across Lago de Maracaibo in search of the Huntington's gene, nearly drowned in a storm.

She used her voice as an instrument in clinic – I often saw it relax ornery patients. Her body language, too, was expressive enough that it could turn the neurological exam, which sick people often feel as invasive scrutiny, into human contact that made her patients feel appreciated. When testing muscle tone, she moved patients' arms and legs in a way that soothed them even as she assessed their deficits.

One of my theories about Anne was that she had a solution to every hospital problem, and I liked to test my theory. Once, I asked her: "Anne, what if I don't get this first grant I'm applying for, and have no money to do research?" When I had put that question to my residency director – the control subject in my test – he had gone into an anxious tailspin. Anne just laughed. "You know I'm descended from WASP robber barons, right?" she said. "That makes me a great fundraiser. If you have no grant money, I'll find some for you." Luckily, I got my grant, but I saw her persuade donors to bail out many other young researchers. Like her unit chiefs, the donors only seemed to like her better after they gave her money – evidence for the Ben Franklin effect, in which people think more highly of you after they have done you a favor.

Another hospital question Anne answered for me was the problem of doctors' tears. In an intensive care unit family meeting, I had told a young woman's husband and school-aged son, with a tearful catch in my voice, that she wouldn't survive her brain hemorrhage. Afterwards, a colleague who had been in the meeting asked if I was all right, and maybe I needed to take some time off? That surprised me; I hadn't felt I had lost control. Later, when I ran into Anne in an elevator, I asked her if it was ok to cry when your patient was dying. "Of course!" she said with her usual certainty. "It's rude not to cry." Then she added a little addendum: "Make sure the tears just well up in your eyes and don't trickle down your cheeks. If your grief is too obtrusive, the patient and the family think they have to take care of you." Her advice seemed like a good approach to empathy in general: we should echo the other person's emotion, not deafen them with our own.

Now, when trainees come to me for help, I try to channel Anne's gifts of listening well and tailoring advice to each person. I can only act like her for a short time, though; soon I relapse into generic advice. When I notice I'm sliding into stock phrases, I break off, give the advisee Anne's phone number, and tell them they will learn more by talking with Anne. Even now, more than a decade after she retired, she still knows exactly which programs the trainee should avoid and which lab heads are truly great mentors. It takes one to know one.

Alice Flaherty, MD, PhD
Departments of Neurology and Psychiatry
Harvard Medical School

Prologue

At 1 a.m., Sunday, January 31, 1999, I was woken by the buzzer at the front door. I heard the banging noises that meant my husband, Jack, and our 19-year-old daughter, Ellen, had returned from a week of neuroscience meetings and skiing in Aspen, Colorado. The hall light went on. Then the thump, thump of Jack carrying their two large, heavy suitcases up the three floors to our bedroom.

"Hi! I'm home!" Jack came over and gave me a kiss and a hug. I was so happy to see him home safely. The next day we planned to celebrate the news that we'd received approval for 50,000 square feet of space to develop an Institute for Neurodegenerative Disease at Massachusetts General Hospital (Mass General). It was a big deal, a project we'd worked on so hard, and we were excited about the work ahead. Jack took off his pants. He sat down and took off his socks. He took off his undies and then his shirt and T-shirt. He slid into bed, naked, next to me. "I think I swallowed a bone."

"Why?" Such a complaint was unusual for him.

"Because I had salmon Friday night and ever since I've had a pain every time I swallow. I almost went to the hospital right from the airport. I guess I'll go tomorrow if it's still bothering me."

"Do you want to go now?" I reached out and felt his forehead for sweat. It was cool. I figured that if the issue was urgent, he would be clammy and sweating.

"No. I'm okay. Maybe some Tums will help." He got a Tums and got back into bed. He tossed and turned but I drifted off to sleep.

Suddenly, I was woken by a loud, ghastly grunting. When I turned, I saw Jack's head was bent forward, his beard on his chest. His arms were stiff and clutching his body. His legs were pulled up slightly. He looked like he was choking but I knew immediately that he was having a heart attack. I jumped up to hit him hard on the chest and then I dragged him off the bed onto the floor so I could get more pressure resuscitating him. His head hit the floor with a 'thunk.' I screamed for Ellen, who came right away from her room to see her dad on the floor. I was naked; Jack was naked. She ran for our phone to call 911 and then she was jumping around on the bed in her pants and a T-shirt, phone to her ear, screaming the operator's instructions.

Jack's mouth tasted good. Every few breaths I breathed into him were followed by a sigh from Jack, which made me think I was making headway. I had to compress his chest repeatedly. It was exhausting. This was it! Holy shit! Can I keep it up until the rescue squad gets here? He's dead! No, he can't be! I'm not going to last.

The buzzer went off and Ellen ran down the three flights to let them in. I was beside myself with fear and fatigue. The rescue squad came gasping up the stairs.

"Go and put some clothes on. We'll take it from here," said the EMT standing closest to me.

I went into the bathroom. There were no clothes in there. I came back out while they were applying defibrillator paddles to shock Jack's heart back into action. I put on some clothes. I could see that

2

nothing was bringing a heartbeat back. They put Jack on a stretcher and were bagging him and pumping on his chest as they took him down the narrow, steep flights of stairs to the front door where there was an ambulance. A policeman took Ellen and me in his squad car and we followed the ambulance to the hospital nearest our house, Massachusetts General Hospital, where Jack and I worked.

By the time Ellen and I got there, Jack was being worked on in the major trauma bay of the emergency room. It was busy, as usual, on an early Sunday morning. A few people who recognized me as the chair of the Mass General Neurology Department nodded hello. I walked behind the curtain of the trauma bay where Jack was. It was crowded with doctors, nurses and others all hovering over him performing the resuscitation process. He was intubated and a ventilator was breathing for him. The doctors pumped on him and injected medications directly into his heart. I stood there for what seemed like an eternity, but it was only minutes. Finally, the lead physician came over to me.

"Nothing we have done has brought any heart rhythm back. The only other thing we can try is to slice open his chest and massage his heart directly."

More than 15 minutes had passed since the attack and during that time there had been no blood supplied to his brain. As a neurologist, I knew all too well what that meant. The chances he would be severely disabled intellectually and physically were way too high, and Jack wouldn't have wanted to survive that way. We had discussed it many times. Just how long do you try? Do you use extraordinary efforts? Both of us felt the same – don't go overboard to save the other and regret it later.

I told them to stop.

Ellen was standing beside me. "Dad is gone," I said. "Saving him is not a possibility." She crumpled up next to me and I hugged her.

One of the senior neurology residents walked by and asked what the matter was, and I motioned to Jack, who was also a Mass

General neurologist. The resident went pale. I was too numb to cry. He asked if he could help and he offered to call Walter Koroshetz, a wonderful colleague who was then the vice-chair of the Neurology Service. I didn't know what to say. Walter wanted to come in. I didn't know what to say. Somebody might as well have hit me over the head with a baseball bat. A nurse came to comfort me. I said I wanted an autopsy. Jack and I had focused our careers on studies of the human brain – both living and after death. We both appreciated the value of the autopsy. I also wanted to know his cause of death. I was instructed to take Jack's jewelry – his watch and wedding ring. Ellen and I were allowed one last visit. The tubes were gone, and he was cleaned up. He was still warm. He still smelled like Jack. He still tasted like Jack. He was dead.

Walter arrived. I could see he too was in shock. We went up to my office. Actually, my assistant Bev Mahfuz's office. I called Jack's dad. He nearly passed out. I called my older daughter, Jessie. How was this possible? Jack was only 51. She had just seen him at Christmas, four weeks earlier. He was so strong and healthy. Jessie said she'd come in the morning.

I called my best friend Nancy Wexler, but her message machine was on. I left the message that Jack was dead. I called Bev. She said she would be in in the morning to notify people. Walter suggested I just go home. He would try to spread the word. He drove Ellen and me home. We went upstairs to my room. It was a mess. Jack had peed on the bed in the final throes. Trash and plastic were all around from the activity of the EMTs.

Ellen and I curled up in bed and tried to doze. No such luck.

At 4 a.m. the phone rang. "This is the New England Organ Bank, and we need to ask you a few questions about your husband. First, how much did he weigh?"

What a completely insensitive first question to ask somebody whose loved one had just died! The conversation deteriorated after that, but I donated every part of him I could think of because I knew that Jack would want to help another life if possible. His brain I donated for research.

But I couldn't sleep. I just lay there – stunned. At five-thirty, I tried Nancy again, leaving her another message. I called Zane Hollingsworth, my good friend and lab manager. He said he and his wife would be over as soon as they could. I tried Julie Porter who worked with Nancy. I told her that Jack was dead and that I needed to find Nancy. She was upset. She knew Jack well. She said she'd try to find Nancy. I called Jack's younger sister Janet and brother Stephen. Each conversation was terribly painful. I called my parents. Time passed slowly. Zane and his wife arrived. They took over calling people for me. All my closest friends were from my lab.

Nancy called. "Anne. Anne. This can't be. I'll be there as soon as I can." By 9 a.m., people started coming over. I don't remember much of the details. I only know that Nancy appeared much sooner than I thought possible. Thank God. She was really the only person who could comfort me. She was the only one who could comfort Ellen. Nancy was a second mother to my daughters. We had all experienced so many joyous and difficult times together in Michigan, California, Venezuela and other places. She was already at the house when Jessie arrived. Nancy worked the crowds of people who were descending on me. I wanted people over. I didn't want to be alone. I vacillated between akinetic and frenetic. I rummaged around and found Jack's love letters. I found videotapes that the lab had made that were hysterically funny. We popped them in the video player. One tape featured Zane telling the lab their assignments from Jack who was 'out of town' – impossible experiments that no one could do. Then they put on tuxedos or dresses and sang "*Stand by Your Jack*."

People immediately began bringing food. The table was set up. Deli platters loaded with cheeses and meats, breads, cookies and pasta salads. Somehow, I was taken care of. I didn't have to do anything. I couldn't even think of eating. I could drink, however, and someone brought me a glass of Jack Daniel's. Flowers also arrived even though I had asked that people give money to the John B. Penney, Jr., MD Memorial Research Fund at Mass General rather than flowers. Soon the apartment was full of them, and their aromas were too strong. For the first time in my memory, the football championship Super Bowl game went by unnoticed that Sunday.

Nancy stayed. I needed somebody to sleep with me the first night. Everything scared me. I tossed and turned and cried and sobbed. Everything was ruined. Jack was everything to me. What could I possibly do? I couldn't imagine life without him.

Jack's sister's husband helped us choose a funeral home. Nancy, Jack's sister and her husband came along and together we chose a modest coffin. We brought clothes for Jack. I had his jeans and one of his favorite Bahama's shirts. We had to bring a sports jacket too because his arm bones and skin had been donated along with his brain and eyes. I had decided I wanted an Irish wake with an open coffin. I knew the undertaker would make Jack look totally normal despite the removal of most organs. Jessie, in particular, wanted to see him again. After the wake, I was going to have him cremated and so I had to pick out an urn for the ashes. The funeral home guy said that anything could be put in the coffin with Jack except golf balls, which tended to explode when the cremation took place.

Wednesday evening, we had the wake. Jack looked so peaceful, almost smiling, in the coffin. Jessie, Ellen and I put all sorts of goodies in with him. The Tolkien books he loved, a little bottle of Jack Daniel's, pictures, goodbye cards and notes and my Swiss Army knife. I kept his knife for myself. Many, many people came to the wake. A long continuous line. I had to endure – trying to communicate. I played Crosby, Stills and

Nash on a boom box. After the wake, we went to Jack's sister's home for dinner with all of Jack's cousins, aunts and uncles. At least, I could have a drink there.

Nancy continued to stay. Thank God. On Thursdays, Neurology Grand Rounds takes place at 9 a.m. in the Ether Dome at Mass General. That week, by coincidence, the New England Organ Bank was scheduled to make an unusual presentation on Organ Donation. Jane Holtz, Neurology's hospital vice-president, was going to be part of the presentation as her daughter had been an organ donor after she was hit by a drunk driver and became brain-dead. The whole thing had a special meaning for me now and I wanted to go and put in my two bits. Also, I wanted to appear at the hospital and give a special message to the department. I discussed it with Nancy, and we decided it was okay if I just went in to give my message and then leave. I couldn't stay through it. I was too restless.

The walk to the hospital was very difficult. Outside, I felt completely vulnerable and very unsafe as if I would be physically hurt. As I approached the hospital, the sirens of ambulances immediately reminded me of Jack's death. I couldn't look at the emergency room when I passed it on the way to the elevators in my building.

In the Ether Dome, I told my department colleagues that I had just been through the worst time of my life. I wanted to thank all of them for their kind support. I also wanted to pass on a piece of advice that meant a lot to me now that Jack was gone. I told them about what my friend, Marilyn Albert, had said to me after her husband had died suddenly in a car accident. In my usual blunt way, I had asked how she could stand not being able to say goodbye. She said she and her husband had had hard times together and that as part of learning to get along despite their differences, they had agreed never to go to bed without reaffirming their love for each other. She could feel sure that he knew she loved him, and he loved her as well. This bit of wisdom was of great help to me now, since after her tragedy, Jack and I decided to take the same approach.

Finally, I asked everyone to support organ donation and to listen closely to the morning presentation. Jack had died outside the hospital and wasn't a candidate for living organ donation, but I wanted them to know that he gave what he could to help other people: his corneas, his brain, his skin, and long bones. I wanted them all to know how important this was.

There! I had given my message. Nancy and I walked home.

My parents arrived from Chicago late Thursday morning and checked into the Omni Parker Hotel just two blocks away from our Beacon Hill apartment. They asked me down to their hotel for lunch. I had to leave my warm and safe apartment and walk outside in the cold. I was afraid to be outside. Nancy wanted to go with me. She knew that I was not close to my parents, and they had never really appreciated Jack. Fortunately, there wasn't too much snow on the frigid street.

When we found my parents in the hotel restaurant, they seemed more interested in the New England clam chowder the Omni Parker was famous for than in how I might be feeling.

"Thank God you work and have a profession to keep you going and financially independent!" said my mother. She showed no sadness or emotion.

"Look at Gammo. My father died when she was still in her forties," said my father.

Gammo was my father's mother. But his comparison seemed tone-deaf. Gammo was 15 years younger than her husband, my grandfather, and their relationship was much more distant than Jack's and mine. My parents were very awkward and tried to put a good face on things but there was no comfort, no warmth. They seemed to think I would magically get through it. They stayed overnight. My mother found it physically difficult to walk up to my apartment and they saw that I had many friends watching over me.

Nancy left the next day. Then Jessie left for the University of Michigan. Then Ellen left for Oberlin College. Zane helped me take Ellen to the airport. I was shaking when I went up to the counter with her. I wondered how I was going to make it without any of them. All I could think of was how much I wanted to be dead too. I wanted to jump off the deck of my apartment. I wanted to drink myself into a deadly stupor and never wake up. I felt as if my insides had fallen out. I had no appetite. I just couldn't go on without Jack. I felt as if I had been skinned alive and I was oozing from the wounds.

Fortunately, friends and neurology residents Jang-Ho Cha, Janice Hayes-Cha, Alice Flaherty, Diana Rosas, Sharin Sakurai and Leslie Shinobu set up a call schedule to make sure someone stayed with me at night. The Night Watch got me through that first acute period. I began to go back to work after about two weeks. I stayed a few hours, spent most of the time looking out the window and then went back home. There I could sit in my living room and have a drink. Flowers arrived and arrived. Each day I got piles of sympathy notes. I read each one and then sorted them in paper bags I kept by my chair – one for the personal ones and a second one for simple sympathy cards. About 7 p.m., my night watch person arrived to spend the night, talk to me and make sure that I was safe.

In the beginning, I felt like I had a bad concussion (and I knew what a concussion felt like). My head was full of sheared Jello and I had trouble latching on to any one thought. If I moved too fast, I felt off-balance. I gradually became more frantic. Everything I thought about led back to Jack. I couldn't get away from it. Work and home. No escape.

Just two weeks earlier, Jack and I had been overjoyed to learn that Mass General had approved our proposal to establish a new center where top researchers could accelerate the search for cures for Parkinson's, Huntington's and other neurodegenerative diseases.

Now everything was ruined. After 28 years of marriage, Jack was everything to me. What could I possibly do? Jack and I had been pretty much inseparable. Work and family, we did everything together as Jack-and-Anne, Anne-and-Jack. He was quiet and content to play a supporting role to my risk-taking, extroverted nature. Together, we had done so much, lived so intensely, worked so hard.

1

• • • • •

A Fascination with Disorderly Movements

I grew up in a big house on a large lot two blocks from Lake Michigan in Winnetka, Illinois. Our house was built on a hill with woods behind us. Off the terrace, another hill went down to the lawn below. A huge elm tree grew outside my window with a swing on a low branch that swung out over the hill above the lawn. I was master of our swing, going way up high and almost flipping over. The Pateras lived next door with five children in a huge old Victorian house. They had a swing that was even bigger – it swung out over the entire bluff. We spent hours taking turns on the swing. Hold on to the ropes. Lean way back and stick your feet out as you accelerate. Tuck in your feet on the return. That way, the swing went more than 30 feet off the ground. The speed, the wind through your hair and the height were exhilarating. As a kid, I had no fear of heights.

The Pateras were among the first in the neighborhood to have a TV in the early 1950s so I spent all my time at their house watching the Mickey Mouse Club, Little Rascals and cartoons. Despite my physical aggressiveness, I was very shy among adults and strangers.

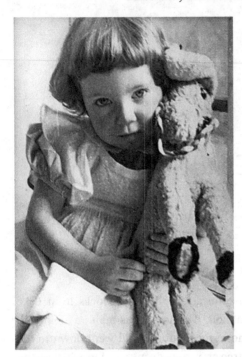

Figure 1.1 Me at three years old.

I was always worried that the Pateras were sick of me. I was sure that nobody really liked me. My mother wanted me to be the cute daughter of her dreams and dressed me up in little dresses, but I wanted to wear my shorts in the dirt and the mud. My father seemed to like me – we raked leaves together, walked up to the hardware store and fixed things – but I wasn't the cute little girl my mother wanted (Figure 1.1).

Ironically, my mother was not exactly happy in the traditional role of housewife and mother that she was expected to play. She had earned her undergraduate degree in physics from Vassar College in 1940 and gave up a promising career in science to marry my father. In college, she wanted to go on to earn a PhD but was discouraged by the Dean of Students. Instead, she was hired to be a human computer at the MIT Radiation Laboratory. She was one of about five women (among 2,000 men) whose job it was to calculate the long division and multiplication problems for the men. At the time, the pocket calculator didn't exist. She usually finished her assignments in the morning and could work on radar development in the afternoon – she had at least three patents on radar development. She was asked to work on the Manhattan Project (the development of the nuclear bomb) at Argonne Laboratories in Chicago but by then she was pregnant with my older brother and couldn't work near radiation. As brilliant and beautiful as she was, she was not a warm mother, and I keenly felt her disappointment in me.

As a little kid, I had a terrible temper that often resulted in screaming tantrums. My parents sent me to my room. But the anger rose up in me as a physical sensation that I was not able to get rid of. After a while the anger eased. But if I got no attention, I stood at the top of the stairs, wailed away, then held my breath until I passed out and tumbled down to the bottom of the stairs.

My middle name is Buckingham and in school I was teased about being a 'bucking Ham.' I was skinny and small with a Buster Brown haircut, but my dad had taught me how to hold my fists and fight. "Haul back and hit them as hard as you can right between the eyes."

I took his advice to heart and in first grade I distinguished myself by hanging out with Wicky and Ned – causing trouble, fighting on the playground and beating up anyone who tried to take my ball, bat or baseball mitt away from me. At the end of the year, Wicky, Ned and I conspired to frown instead of smile when the class picture was taken. Apparently, they lost their nerve because when the photograph came back, I was the only one frowning.

Only later did I learn to be proud to be descended from the Buckinghams – a spirited, enterprising family of pioneers who arrived from England in 1637. (The other families of my ancestors came from England in 1637 (the Chandlers), France in 1655 and Switzerland in 1710.) Five generations later, Ebenezer Buckingham, his wife and 10 of their 13 children moved to the Muskingum River in Ohio in 1799 just as the Northwest Territory was opening up. The large family became farmers and learned to hunt the local game. After the autumn harvest, the five Buckingham brothers cut down some of the abundant oaks and black walnut trees, fashioned them into a good-sized raft, loaded it up with local produce and floated down the Ohio and Mississippi rivers all the way to New Orleans. There, they sold the goods and walked back home along the Natchez Trace to their farm. The second year they did this, they bought letters of credit from New York banks in New Orleans. They then took a steamer to New York and cashed in the letters at a handsome profit. They walked home. Finally, in the third year they went to New York again, bought horses and rode home.

This group of brothers were entrepreneurs and explorers. The oldest brother, Ebenezer, started a trading post. In the 1840s, brothers Alvah and Ebenezer Buckingham walked to Chicago where they found commerce in the city from boats coming down Lake Michigan. Alvah and Ebenezer went home and persuaded the other brothers to come look at bustling Chicago – the population was still less than 10,000 but the Union Pacific Railroad was expected to come soon. Surely, it was an exciting place, an opportunity. The other brothers were not impressed. They thought Chicago was a swamp and not good for farming and went home to Ohio.

But Alvah and his brother-in-law, Solomon Sturges, went to Chicago and in 1855 they built the first grain elevator. They bought grain in late summer as it came in on trains from the west, stored up to 70,000 bushels in their huge grain elevator buildings over the winter and sold it in the spring at a huge profit. They built bigger grain storage elevators – enough to hold 700,000 bushels of grain – in the next few years. The Buckinghams became early leaders in Chicago. They used their wealth to build, among other things, the

Buckingham fountain and donated many works of art to the Art Institute of Chicago.

Meanwhile, the Ohio side of the Buckinghams continued to farm. When I was born my mother suggested naming me after her grandmother, Anna Buckingham. My father piped up and said that *his* grandmother was Anna Buckingham! It turned out the women were not the same person. My father was a descendant of Alvah Buckingham and my mother was a descendant of Alvah's brother, Milton. That was when my parents realized that they were fourth cousins.

I like to think I've inherited the curiosity and enterprising spirit of the Buckinghams. Maybe that was why I rebelled against many of the expectations of the upper-class society the family had embraced by the time I came along.

Much to my mother's chagrin, I spent a lot of my childhood outside playing baseball, climbing trees, starting fires, building forts in the woods and damming up the brooks and gutters after big rains. There was a small park a few hundred feet from our house and the neighborhood kids played pickup baseball incessantly. I loved to play and was good at it. I had a strong throw, and I could hit well enough to get on base consistently.

Summers, my parents brought the family to visit my grandmother on her farm in Ohio, and when I was six I learned that cornsilk was good to smoke. My father smoked a pipe and he got me a corncob pipe and taught me how to pick the best silk off the ends of the ears of corn in the field. He puffed on his tobacco and I puffed on my corncob pipe. Before going home, I stashed away a bunch of cornsilk in a brown lunch bag to take back to Winnetka. I went up to the local grocery store, 'Poulopoulos,' and got a popsicle and then pulled out a cornsilk stogie and smoked it. The housewives from Winnetka were appalled. Even that young, I enjoyed shocking them.

In elementary school, I had difficulty reading. I could only read by saying the words in my mind. As school went on, I never gained speed. Words were patterns of black and white and had no meaning unless I said them aloud in my head. But I liked reading. I woke up early and could read in the mornings when it was quiet before anyone else was up. I loved *Heidi* about a little girl in Switzerland living high in the mountains with her grandfather during the summers. Maybe someday I could live in my own tiny cabin. I wanted to be like Pippi Longstocking who was marvelously scrappy and rebellious and did things on her own terms. I wanted to read faster, but I never exceeded more than about 20 pages an hour. Every year, there were standardized reading tests, and I could never get more than halfway through the test. My reading level was always a couple of grades behind. I did well in other subjects, so I never received any special help. Dyslexia only started being diagnosed clinically in the 1970s.

I excelled, however, in outdoor activities. The street we lived on was a dead end at the top of the bluff. Snake Hill. In the winter, the hill became the best sledding hill in town and people came from all over. We neighborhood kids iced it down to improve the sledding. I could go down the hill at top speed standing on my Flexible Flyer, drop down to a lying position and do a 360 turn. We built tunnels of snow to sled through. Once in a while, someone injured him/herself running into a telephone pole, but we were lucky enough to avoid injury.

In elementary school, most of my friends were boys. In fourth grade, the gym teacher declared that I had to play with the girls. After two innings and several home runs, he realized that I was better off with the boys, and I was allowed back with my friends. Even though I was small, all the boys learned I was not to be messed with as I hauled off and slugged them if they picked on me. Since I thought my life depended on it, I wouldn't hold anything back. Perhaps this was why I was later unfazed by the male-dominated culture of medical school. I already knew how to beat them at their own game.

I didn't feel like a typical girl, but I never doubted that I was one or wanted to be a boy. I felt like my own, singular self – like Pippi Longstocking. I was never comfortable joining the little groups of girls who seemed to be always gossiping about somebody or conspiring to do someone in. But I never had a fistfight with a girl. I was in the Brownies and the Girl Scouts but hated it – not only the cute little projects we were made to do but also most of the other little girls, whom I perceived as wimpy. That attitude too was something I carried with me as an adult. I could never identify with feminists who complained about unfair treatment when the obvious solution seemed to be to figure out a way to be treated fairly or at least get what you want. I had no intention to be one of the boys but I knew their game. I also didn't want to be one of the girls. I was able to escape from the Girl Scouts with the help of one of the friends I'd managed to make there. One day when my friend had volunteered to bring in the Kool-Aid and cookies and walked by, I stuck out my foot. In an instant my friend, the Kool-Aid and the cookies were all over the floor. I was overjoyed when my mother received a call from the Scoutmaster kicking me out.

Despite or because of how active I was as a kid I was also aware from an early age of illness and how the body could have trouble moving. My aunt, my mother's sister, was paralyzed from the waist down as the result of a car accident. Although I can't remember ever seeing her, I could imagine her in a wheelchair. I always took care not to step on cracks because I thought it would break *my* mother's back.

Then in the spring of 1951, when I was four, my mother came down with polio. Actually, our whole family got sick with polio, but we just got the 'stomach flu' while my mother developed excruciating muscle pain and weakness. The polio virus causes fever, nausea and vomiting. But in some people, it infects the muscle and from there the virus crosses into the nerves that control the muscles and travels up the motor nerves to the spinal cord where it kills the nerve cells.

My mother was in bed quite a while and eventually weakness settled permanently into her right lower leg. She was able to walk but never again could she stand on her tiptoes on the right.

I also drew strength from the farming side of my family, and in particular my grandmother, Elsie Bishop Buckingham, who'd married a Buchwalter named Morris. The Buchwalters were Mennonites who'd emigrated to the US from Switzerland in 1710, migrated to central Ohio in about 1800 and farmed the land. The farm in Hallsville is 300 acres of land that stretches about a mile down to the 'bottom' land. The soil is dark and rich. When the family settled there, they planted an apple orchard and named the farm 'Applethorpe Farm.' When I was a kid, the farm had a herd of about twenty Herefords, six milk cows, ten to fifteen sows and fields of corn, wheat, oats, soybeans and hay. There were several barns. The farmhouse had a well with a pump for drinking water. An icehouse and smokehouse still existed when I was six or seven.

The summers we spent at my grandmother's farm fed my curiosity and love of nature (Figure 1.2). My older brother, Peyton, my younger sister, Lisa, and I trapped snapping turtles, flew homemade four-foot-high box kites in the pasture and hunted arrowheads in the corn fields (Figure 1.3). Alice and Earl Fox lived on the farm and ran the day-to-day activities, and from them I learned to milk the cows before breakfast and ride on the running board of Earl's pickup truck down to the field to feed corn to the pigs.

I rode on the tractors and the wagons as they plowed the corn or soybeans, harvested the wheat and cut the hay. The smells at the farm are settled into my memory – the old farmhouse and barn filled with hay, the milking shed below, the cows, the calves, the hogs and the piglets, manure, sitting in the wagons of wheat, oats and hay.

My grandmother, Ganny, had never learned to drive but had to after my grandfather's death. I remember her taking us into Chillicothe, the nearest city about half an hour away, and weaving

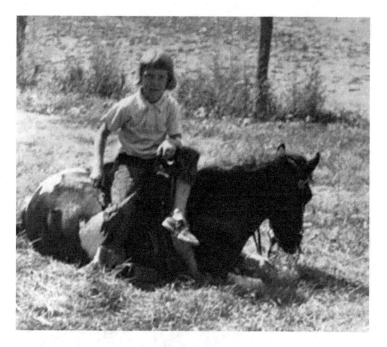

Figure 1.2 Me on a pony at our farm in Ohio.

along the road. It was both scary and fun to ride with her as she drove up and down the hills in the middle of the road – almost like riding on a roller coaster. Ganny was easy to get along with and always seemed to have a smile on her face. She never got cross and called us 'little creatures.' Ganny was enterprising. During the Depression of the 1930s, she offered to take the daughters of rich Ohio families to study in Switzerland at the American School for two years and travel through Europe. Her compensation covered all costs for her own two daughters and herself. The trip provided a first-class education for my mother and my aunt.

At the farm, I spent a lot of time just watching what was happening before me. I spent hours inspecting the ants on the ivy

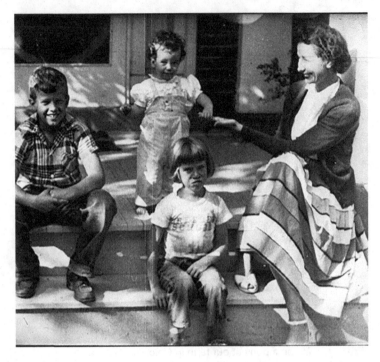

Figure 1.3 Me with Peyton, Lisa and Mother.

growing across the screen on my bedroom window. The ants traveled up and down the vine and were shepherds tending to small round bugs I later learned were called aphids. The ants milked the aphids' nectar and kept them safe by taking them back to the nest at night.

At other times, I wandered into the pasture where our herd of cattle was grazing. I squatted on the ground and waited quietly. The cows gradually approached and sniffed the grass near me. They were big and I was small. Their breath was warm and sweet-smelling, and I was only a little afraid. In the pig field, it was a different matter. The big sows were potentially dangerous, and

I was told to stay behind the fence, where I watched intently. That was when I first developed what became a lifelong attachment and even identification with piglets. The little piglets were the most fun! They were born in litters of 8-10 and several litters ran around the field together. Not only were they incredibly cute but watching them I saw that they played tag! One little piglet ran at the group and singled out someone to butt. The whole group then split up, running in all directions, and the pig who'd been butted had to tag the next one. The games went on for a long time. All this fascinated me.

One night at the farm, as my parents came to bed, they checked on me as they did every night. As they approached the room, they heard a cry and a thud. They opened the door to find me on the floor with a large gash over my eye. I had been dreaming I was a dive-bomber airplane and had catapulted myself headfirst off the bed into the dresser. I was taken in the middle of the night into Chillicothe for my first stitches. I remember the bright white light and green color of the cloth curtains. The lidocaine stung but numbed the area. Then I felt a tug with each stitch. I had a large bandage covering my left eyebrow. The next day it hurt but it was worth it to show my friends my wound when I got back to Winnetka. Having stitches is one of the milestones of childhood and I had reached it without any serious damage.

Every grade, I was switched to a new class because I was a troublemaker. I talked too much in class, passed notes, kicked kids under the chair and started fights at recess. Each year, the school hoped I would behave better with a new set of friends. Unfortunately, I just made more friends in each class and didn't improve my troublemaking.

Outside of school, I was made to go to dancing school, which I hated because I had to put on a dress and white socks and patent leather shoes. I did my best to sulk in a chair and avoid dancing with the little boys who also obviously didn't want to be there either. I did like boys though and in fifth grade I spent many afternoons making out on the beach with Danny or Peter.

My brother taught me how to shoplift. We had jackets that had an elastic band around the waist and zipped up the front.

"Just be cool," my brother said. "You have to show confidence – not nervousness or guilt. Browse through the comic books and slip one into your jacket. You can do the same with candy bars and gum."

It was so simple, and we soon had a huge stash. We couldn't eat it all. Then Halloween came and we had so much candy we didn't know what to do, so we buried it in the woods.

Then there was the time a bunch of us, including my brother, Peyton, were playing in the woods at the top of the bluff and found an old steel wheel with the tire still on it. We decided to roll it down the bluff into the trees above our neighbor's house to see how far it could go. We hadn't counted on the weight of its hub, which increased its acceleration. We all stood there and watched as the wheel careened into the trees and then were amazed as it kept going across the flat roof of the neighbor's garage and onto the roof of Mr. Webster's antique model Roadster. The roof and hood of the car were crushed.

That night at dinner my parents told us how the poor Websters' antique car had been destroyed by vandals rolling a wheel down the hill. My brother kicked me under the table, and I tried to keep a straight face. That night I couldn't sleep. I was a shoplifter and now, as I lay awake, I felt hopelessly guilty and bad to think I was becoming a thief and a vandal! Finally, I cried out and my mother came into my room. I confessed everything – the shoplifting and the destruction of the car. I told her I was sorry and I'd try to work to make it up.

My brother was furious. What a worthless little tattletale I was. My mother took us up to the stores and made us confess to the management and pay for the estimated cost of the stolen goods out

22

of our allowances going forward. We had to do volunteer work for the Websters, although we couldn't possibly pay them back for the car. Fortunately, they had somewhat of a soft spot for us, perhaps because they had no children of their own. It was a defining moment for me. I vowed never to steal again or hurt people who didn't deserve it.

In sixth grade, my parents decided to send me to private school. The Winnetka public schools were very good but huge and my parents were afraid I would be lost in the large classes. I was devastated to think of switching schools and leaving my old friends for what we called, 'North Shore Country Day where all the fairies go and play.' Ultimately, it was a good decision. In the public school system, I would not have been challenged academically because I always scored poorly on the standardized tests used to determine placement levels. Private school gave me more academic support.

Going to NSCD was pivotal too because that was where I made a new group of friends, boys and girls, including Les Moore, who became my best friend. Les had four older brothers and sisters who were all very popular in school – intellectuals, activists and athletes. Her mother continued to run her husband's business after his death from alcohol-induced liver failure when Les was six. After school, Les and I walked the two miles to her house and went up to a room above the garage to play poker and smoke cigarettes. On the weekends, I hung out at Les' house, along with her older siblings and their friends, and that was an education, too.

Middle school was relatively uneventful. I played field hockey, basketball and baseball. I got through my classes. I had several boyfriends, one of whom taught me how to whistle really loudly without using my fingers. I was still punching people who did me wrong. In sixth grade, when a boy grabbed the basketball from me one day in the gym, I slugged him right between the eyes so

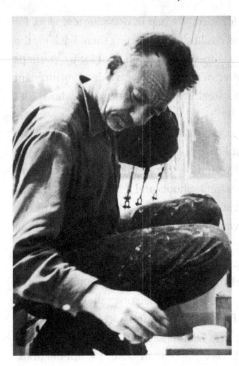

Figure 1.4 My father, Hobart P. Young, Jr.

hard his nose bled. I got the ball back, but my hand was sore and throbbing and later it swelled up and turned black and blue.

That evening, I showed my swollen hand to my dad (Figure 1.4). Would my hand go back to normal? When my dad asked what had happened and I told him how I'd punched a boy bigger than me because he stole my basketball, I could see my dad's eyes light up with pride. His 'Tiger Annie' had prevailed.

My dad liked to do watercolor and pen drawings of landscapes and I used to sit next to him and draw as well. He taught me about mixing colors, perspective, clouds, light and shadows. My skill later developed into the ability to doodle and draw cartoons. Cartoons depend on people's postures and distinguishing characteristics. They are a wonderful way to express your feelings.

I have loved to ski ever since I learned in our backyard on the bluff using my mother's wooden skis with bear-trap bindings. I loved the speed and throwing myself off jumps. Initially, I had no fear. I hated the poles, so I didn't use them. In middle school, we traveled to the local ski areas in Wisconsin – an hour away. We held on to the rope tow going up the tiny hills and going down I made sure to speed. My classmates and I set up jumps. It was exhilarating to lift off the jump, hands in the air, and fly.

But the time we went skiing at Iron Mountain with Mr. Steele, our eighth-grade teacher, changed me. Mr. Steele also skied without poles. That day he came down the mountain and hit the dip of an access road with too much speed. He flipped up and over and landed on his head, crushing a cervical vertebra. He had to be in a 'halo' brace for months. After that, I began to fear skiing. I began using poles and never again had that exhilarating feeling of flying except in my dreams.

Everybody was maturing before I did. I was young for my class, but even so, I was a late bloomer. In the girls' locker room, everybody was wearing bras, and I was still in my undershirt. I wanted to disappear. My mother was singularly unhelpful and in addition my pride was such that I never asked her what to expect. My friends taught me how to shave my legs and under my arms. I was a stinky little kid. My father was a strict believer in the beauty of sweat and BO and said anyone who used deodorant was some sort of fairy. And as far as I could tell, my mother didn't sweat. She always smelled sweet and nice. She had naturally curly dark hair and wore a tiny amount of makeup and powder. She was actually rather beautiful (Figure 1.5).

I felt awkward and lumpy and ugly and tried to compensate by being tough. I was always being a wise-off in class. My grades weren't particularly good either, so in my sophomore year of high school, my parents decided to start paying me for good grades. They later told me they felt very guilty about doing this, but they were

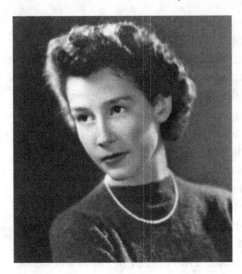

Figure 1.5 My mother, Louise Buchwalter Young.

worried I was just going to goof off and then not get into a good college. I loved the deal. An "A" was $25 bucks. My grades shot up and I got a lot of money.

I continued to excel in sports. I liked to run, play ball, ski, and ride the waves in Lake Michigan. I played fullback on the junior varsity and varsity field hockey teams. Even though I was 5′6″ and 115 pounds, I could scare the pants off a forward or halfback from any other team. I had sheer determination and had learned to never show any doubt. Our team finished high school unbeaten *and* unscored upon.

Basketball was the sport that obsessed me, though. From middle school on, I was the outside shooter and by high school I was captain of the varsity basketball team. When I was a freshman in high school, I played the position of "rover" – the player who could cross the centerline, cover the rover from the other team and set up the offense. Later all players played full court. Les Moore was a forward and was great one-on-one to the basket. We collaborated. I practiced the outside shots from the top of the key, but if there was any hope of a break, I passed the ball to her and she went to the basket. We won most of the games. I had a final year average of twenty points per game. My overhead shots swished from the top of the key. Les always beat me to the basket. I was the queen of the outside shot. I spent endless hours shooting, trying to perfect it.

In high school, I was interested in science and art. Two classmates and I were given the opportunity to visit the University of Chicago School of Medicine for a one-day introduction to medicine. I didn't want to see actual surgery because I was frightened by blood, so I signed up to see a demonstration of immunity in mice. I figured I'd be fine with little mice. A group of us stood around the doctor and watched as he pulled out a live white mouse, bent it to the side and quickly shaved the hair off the abdomen. He pointed out the liver pressing against the skin. He then picked up a full 50 ml syringe (about the size of the mouse) with a large needle. As he brought the needle close to the mouse, my vision went yellow and the next thing I remember is the crowd of students and the doctor staring down at me lying flat on my back on the linoleum floor. I had fainted dead away. It took about half an hour to recover but I remember nothing of the rest of the day. It was clear to me, however, that I could lose consciousness quickly and unexpectedly at any time. I couldn't imagine being a doctor.

My father had been a chemistry major in college and my mother had been a physics major. They were very interested in science and talked about issues like gravity and the origin of the universe at the dinner table. Together, they liked to design experiments at home. They made a self-maintaining terrarium and a new style of fluorescent Christmas tree decorations illuminated by a blacklight. They measured ozone levels with a contraption my father made to fit in the sunroof of our car and tried to produce cold fusion in our backyard.

Issues of *Science*, *Scientific American*, *National Geographic* and *Natural History* were always on the coffee table in our living room. I liked to flip through the magazines and look at the pictures and sometimes read the articles. I was fascinated by biological studies. One article on planaria particularly fascinated me. The scientists were able to show that the little planaria flatworms could learn to go through a maze to get a reward. This on its own was surprising but even more amazing was that if the trained planaria were ground up and fed to untrained planaria, the novice planaria learned the maze instantly. Could you really eat another animal's memories and acquire them yourself? I wondered whether amphetamine or other drugs let the planaria learn even faster.

Our high school organized activities to raise social awareness. Some of us signed up to go to the Chicago State Mental Hospital on Tuesday nights to visit with and entertain the inpatients in the locked male ward. On the dreary winter evening bus rides, I often sat with my friend, Stetson Ames, as we rode in the dark down Irving Park Road. Stets had been the new boy in class in eighth grade. He was tall and cute. We shared classes in German and advanced mathematics – calculus. We danced at the parties and sat in class together. We were on-and-off boyfriend and girlfriend.

This was the first time I saw people with neuropsychiatric disorders. The ward was a dreary, colorless, smelly place – a building with one huge room and a domed ceiling and beds all around the periphery. There were tall windows on both sides. The floor was cement and patients walked the room, sometimes peeing in the corners, many with what I later learned was tardive dyskinesia – their tongues moving in and out, their lips smacking, their faces grimacing. They paced the floors. Wanting to lighten things up, we brought in a phonograph and played records with the latest popular songs – *He's So Fine* by the Chiffons, *Little*

Surfer Girl by the Beach Boys, *My Boyfriend's Back* by the Angels. We could get some people to dance and others to talk. That human beings could suffer in this way made my suburban life feel complacent and coddled. When I went home, I scolded my parents for being uncaring hypocrites who squandered their lives away in business, social life and suburbia. Why didn't they use their intellect to do something more positive for the world?

Whether I had any influence or not, I have no idea. In my sophomore year in high school, my mother started putting together a series of books for adult education on various aspects of the universe (Figure 1.6).

Then in my senior year, she began writing and publishing popular science books: *Power Over People, Blue Planet, Earth's Aura, The Unfinished Universe* and *Islands.* She had finally found a way to channel her intellect to educate the public about the universe. She continued to write into her eighties. She wanted to be the Rachel Carson of physics.

Unlike my parents and their friends, Mrs. Moore was a staunch advocate of the civil rights movement and helped organize support for African Americans in Chicago. We often sat at her feet on the rug in her living room while she discussed politics and current events. Les and I were the youngest, but we liked to sit around and listen, as folk music by people like Woody Guthrie, Lead Belly, Joan Baez and Bob Dylan played in the background. Les' oldest brother Phil was a Freedom Marcher in Mississippi in 1963 and was arrested and beaten. Mrs. Moore also experienced violence when she went to Alabama for the famous march from Selma to Montgomery led by Martin Luther King to protest White Southerners' resistance to the newly legislated voting rights for African Americans. In July of 1965, Mrs. Moore was one of several women who arranged for Martin Luther King to give a talk on the Village Green in Winnetka, Illinois. This was not a popular move

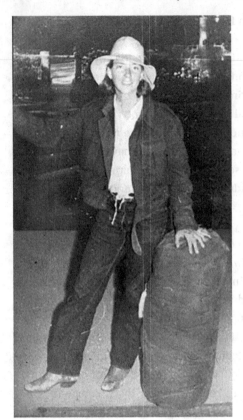

Figure 1.6 Me returning from camp in Arizona at age 15.

at the time when Winnetka flagrantly discriminated against all minorities who tried to buy houses and move in.

In the summers, I often visited Les in Charlevoix, Michigan where the Moores had a summer house on Lake Charlevoix in the northern lower peninsula. It was a large, rustic place with screened sleeping porches on each side – one for the girls, the other for the boys. We water-skied, played card games like Bridge and War, rode horses and goofed off. One summer near the end of high school, Les and I and several friends took the horses overnight up to a back pasture. We set up camp and made a fire. Les pulled out several bottles of whiskey and rum and we drank until we were reeling around and unable to stand up. We finished off all the bottles and passed out. The next day we felt like shit, but eventually, having survived our first drunk, we rode the horses home.

2
• • • • •

Chemistry Major at All Women's College

On September 10, 1965, I took the train from Chicago to Vassar College in Poughkeepsie, New York. I'd wanted to go to Radcliffe where Les Moore's older sister went and because my brother was a student at Harvard, but I didn't get in. I was accepted to Vassar and Mount Holyoke. My mother had gone to Vassar, but I chose it because the students seemed diverse and fun to talk to when I visited.

The housing office had assigned me to a two-person double – one little room for the bunk beds and another for studying. I was frightened to meet my roommate. I had never roomed with anyone, and I liked to be by myself in my room.

My roommate opted to occupy the small inside room and I got the big outside room. For the first two months, I rarely saw my roommate, who holed herself up in the room. Smoke emanated from under the door. I had never smelled the aroma before. It wasn't tobacco or cornsilk. It was pungent and slightly spicy. In November, she was thrown out.

I now had two rooms to myself. It was great. I played bridge with several others in the dorm. But mostly I stayed to myself. I went to classes every day. I played basketball and two of the older teammates invited me out to drink a few beers at the local pub. I was only 17 and so I couldn't order but they got an extra few beers for me. We struck up a great friendship. Pigeon Orrick was the master of the inside *and* outside shot and Mary Donneally was a great defense player. I fit right in playing the interface between offense and defense. Our team won most games and when Pigeon asked if I wanted to join the neighborhood Poughkeepsie basketball team sponsored by the local Arlington Sporting Goods shop, I said sure. We played in a downtown gym near the Brown Derby bar. The three of us, along with the other women on the team from the local community college faculty, trashed every team in the region.

Pigeon encouraged me to go down to New York City and visit my former roommate.

"She probably has some great dope."

"Dope?"

"Yeah. Dope. Marijuana. She was always smoking the best." Ah. That was the smell from under her door.

I got on the train to New York City and went to my former roommate's apartment. The 23rd floor. She came to the door and invited me in. It was a wide-open, modern apartment with floor to ceiling windows looking out over the city. Her parents were in the living room. She led me to her bedroom and closed the door. She rolled a big joint.

"But your parents are home," I said.

She said that her parents were always trying to steal her dope and we had nothing to worry about. We smoked a joint and I thought, "This is stupid. I don't feel anything." Then I bought three ounces from her and went back down to the street. The walk to Grand Central Station was like going through a time warp. Everything slowed down. I was hungry. I felt slightly disoriented and giddy but satisfied. Somehow, I got on the train back to Poughkeepsie. Everything was weird. The colors and sounds and tastes and smells were all so vivid. Time was distorted. But it was so fun and relaxing.

I became a small-time dope dealer. I was a privileged white girl whose parents gave me an allowance for the whole semester at once, so I had cash reserves; I could stock up and then sell dope to my friends at a small profit. In December, I turned 18, the legal drinking age in New York. Every night we'd hit the bars around 11 p.m. and I'd set up four beers before they had last call at midnight. Thursday night we'd start earlier, and, on the weekend, we'd get stoned and drunk and bar hop down the Poughkeepsie streets. Often, we ended up at the Brown Derby where there was an interracial, raucous crowd and frequent fights. One night, a guy got particularly ornery, and the police came. He was lean and muscular; the police were overweight and slow. The guy gave five of them the fight of their lives before he was finally subdued with billy clubs and gun butts. At that time, I didn't view law enforcement positively. The cops. Like so many people did at that time, we called them the pigs.

My friends and I crashed the mixers at Vassar. Proper entrance required wearing a skirt, but we wore jeans by sneaking in from the adjacent snack shop. We hung out behind all the guys waiting at the table where they were distributing quarts of beer. The guys all had on sports jackets or West Point uniforms, and if you were clever you could reach between the jackets and snitch a quart of beer, retreat to the corner and drink it. One morning after a Vassar–Yale mixer I woke up to find crumbs of a Baby Ruth candy bar in bed with me and sprinkled across the floor to the door. Evidence of the munchies but no recollection about what had actually happened. Later that morning, I got a call during breakfast from some guy who said he was Andy. He had such a great time with me the night before, he wanted to know if I'd visit him the next weekend. I mumbled something in reply. I had no idea who this Andy was or what we'd talked about. My first alcohol-induced blackout.

34

A group of us used to monopolize one table in the back of the dorm dining room. You had to wear a skirt to dinner but we either threw on a skirt over our jeans or just ignored the rules. We smoked and ate food off each other's plates and trays. People soon learned that sitting at our table could be a difficult experience. We were called the Pigs. The Pig Table. We began to flaunt it. We got Irish coins with pigs on them and wore them around our necks. I remembered how I'd loved watching the pigs play at my grandmother's farm. We rustled up cute passages about pigs, including this one from Nathaniel Hawthorne:

> A drove of pigs passing at dusk. They appeared not so much disposed to ramble and go astray from the line of march as in daylight, but kept together in a pretty compact body. There was a general grunting, not violent at all, but low and quiet, as if they were expressing their sentiments among themselves in a companionable way. Pigs, on a march, do not subject themselves to any leader among themselves, but pass on, higgledy-piggledy, without regard to age or sex. (Nathaniel Hawthorne, journal entry, August 31, 1838)

A perfect description of us Pigs. Expressing our sentiments among ourselves in a companionable way without any leader and keeping together higgledy-piggledy. We painted cute little pink pigs on sheets and used them as tablecloths on special occasions. I had a VW bug that I named Piglet and decorated with little pink pig decals. We pigs were experts at starting food fights. Putting a glob of food on a spoon, I held the bottom end of the spoon just below the edge of the table, put a finger on the tip of the spoon and flung it. I got a nice trajectory, and nobody noticed that I had thrown anything. Once I landed a piece of Jello right next to a guest speaker who was having dinner at our dorm.

In the spring of my freshman year, my parents said that I had to be a debutante.

"Being a debutante is against my principles," I yelled over the dorm phone in the hall outside my room. "I don't intend to be auctioned off like a cow and I certainly don't see any value in being introduced to a group of clueless, eligible males!"

"Being a debutante has nothing to do with those things!" my mother replied calmly. "It's a tradition of social distinction. Your family helped found Chicago and your grandmothers are expecting you to be a debutante. If you say you won't be one, that would be a huge insult to them."

"I don't care." I stomped my foot. "I think it's a disgusting deprecation of females and a waste of money!"

My mother sighed. I could hear her thinking about what to say next. Good thing she didn't know about my pot-dealing or bar-hopping. I was still fist fighting and I wasn't going to stop all the good fun of being bad. Finally, she said what she'd probably been prepared to say all along. "We have tried all our lives to provide you with the best. And if you won't reciprocate and agree to being a debutante, then we will just have to withdraw support for your education."

Now it was my turn to be silent. I thought about suffering through a few dinner dances and a few teas and even a few disgusting events like the Cotillion versus not continuing college or graduating college with a huge debt. I caved. I decided to take the easy road and be a debutante – for my grandmothers and for a free education.

It was really unpleasant. That summer, back in Winnetka, invitations arrived from other debutantes for little parties and teas with elderly ladies and I had to respond formally, on special stationery and in my best handwriting. I tried to refuse as many as I could. I had to shop for dresses to wear to the parties. I had a short waist and nothing ever fit. I always felt humiliated. The few parties that I went to were to appease my parents. I reluctantly put on a dress and appeared. I usually stayed in the corner, drank if possible and went home as soon as I could.

It was all a lead-up to the Cotillion in December that was held at a fancy Chicago hotel. It was supposed to be a charity fundraiser;

only families who could afford the required donations to the Northwestern Memorial Hospital were invited. I went to the Cotillion escorted by my father, my cousin David and a high school boyfriend. David had lived with my family for most of high school after his mother died. He was the most handsome guy imaginable – all the high school girls had come to me to try to get to him. I was allowed two male dates and I figured I'd covered that well. The guys all wore black tails, white shirts with a white bow tie and a carnation in their lapel. Like the other girls, I wore a nice satin gown and white gloves above the elbows, but I had persuaded my mother to let me wear my hair in pigtails. Most of the other girls had complicated hairdos they'd fussed over at the beauty parlor. My mother acquiesced but insisted that I have a silver clasp for each pigtail.

Back at school after winter break, I was no longer myself. Sneaking into mixers with my friends and going out for beers after basketball was no longer fun. *Rubber Soul* had come out and I stayed in my room playing the album over and over. I didn't know why I felt so bad. It was as if I'd swallowed a poisonous potion that was draining all hope from my being. But it was confusing because I also felt very angry and all-powerful. My body was full of energy like it had been as a child when I stood at the top of the stairs and hurled myself down. Now I wanted to pull entire trees out by their roots and grab people by the neck, choke them, throw them to the ground and stomp on their faces. Where did these impulses come from? They scared me, too.

Violent thoughts and images began to spontaneously infiltrate my mind. I spent a lot of time thinking about the sniper who had been all over the news that summer. In what was then the biggest mass shooting in US history, ex-marine Charles Whitman had shot and killed 15 people and injured 31 from his perch on top of a tower at the University of Texas. Most people were understandably shocked and outraged, but when I let my mind go I could almost imagine how powerful he must have felt in those hours before he was shot dead by the police. Whitman had certainly made people stop and take notice.

Alone in my room, my thoughts went something like this: Life was precious and short, but everybody I saw seemed to be way too complacent about their lives. Wasn't there a way to end the pain and suffering in the world? I know it sounds deranged, but my idea was that more random killings would wake people up to value their life more. I fantasized about hooking an automatic rifle up on a roof, aiming it at a busy street corner and rigging it to go off randomly – say, triggered by gamma rays hitting a Geiger counter. More and more I felt like I was losing control. Mornings, I lay in bed and thought about sticking a knife into my heart. I imagined blood spurting out of my chest as I died. The truth is, I hated myself. Retrospectively, I realize I was suffering from a major mood disorder for which I was later treated.

Then, one morning, I was at the coffee shop with some friends and was overcome by a complete and total panic. I ran outside screaming. My friends raced after me and when they caught up and got a hold of me, they forced me to go to the little health center on campus. The nurse there locked me in a room. I sat on my bed reading. The food was terrible, and I was given medication.

After a while, the psychiatrist came in and asked me what the problem was. I stared at my hands in my lap and said nothing. He asked if I was having problems with my family or school. Maybe it was a boyfriend? He sat in a vinyl armchair tapping his foot as he waited for an answer.

Again, I said nothing.

After a couple of days, it was clear that I wasn't going to get out of the health center unless I talked. So, I told the psychiatrist the truth: I wanted to kill people.

He tried to remain impassive, but I saw him startle. Now it was his turn to say nothing. Finally, he asked, "What do you want to do in life?"

"I want to be a doctor."

"That's a bad idea," he frowned. "My advice is: take a long vacation. Take some time off from school."

This was not what I wanted to hear. I wanted to know how I could feel better and stop losing control of my mind. "I thought you were supposed to help me. How is quitting school going to help me?" This was my first encounter with the mental health system and this was singularly unhelpful.

It was hopeless to talk to him. Why had I even tried? I fell back into silence.

I don't know why the health staff finally let me out, but they did. If there was one thing I knew, it was that I wasn't going to see a psychiatrist again. Besides, in those days, seeing a psychiatrist was a stigma that was not much talked about. Having to do so meant a person was seriously crazy. I thought I was just going through a rough spot. By the spring, my depression, which had lasted for months, gradually stopped on its own. This was not the last time I would be depressed.

I was definitely changing. I was no longer the fearless skier who sped down the slope without poles and felt exhilarated. Later that same year, while driving Piglet from Chicago to Poughkeepsie, I had my first panic attack. One minute I was driving on a bright and sunny strip of the Pennsylvania Turnpike and the next minute I was in a tunnel, in the dark. The headlights from oncoming cars shone into my eyes. Trucks and cars zoomed by me, and I saw there was no pullout lane should something go wrong. The world was closing in. My heart was pounding. I needed air. I opened the window, but I had trouble seeing because everything was covered by yellow gauze. I slowed down to about 20 miles an hour and I thought I was going to pass out. Trucks honked and continued to whoosh by at high speed, but I made it to the other end of the tunnel. As soon as I could, I pulled over to the side of the road. It took half an hour before I felt calm enough to drive again. This was my first panic attack. From that point on, I had to avoid tunnels, bridges and highways with no pullout lane.

Meanwhile, it was the 1960s. Beatniks traded in their berets and pipes for tie-dye shirts and bell bottoms and became hippies. The assassinations of Martin Luther King and Bobby Kennedy in 1968 fueled my liberal civil rights and antiwar attitudes.

I spent summers in Chicago working at local hospitals, and on the weekends, I joined Les and others in civil rights marches that went to bigoted, segregated Chicago neighborhoods like Cicero. We were marching for freedom. Fortunately, none of the stones and bottles that people threw at us hit me and I came out of it unscathed. Emotionally, however, I was amazed and angered at the hate people spewed toward others who were different from them. I felt strongly about supporting equal rights and opportunities for all people. As I spent time in the poorer neighborhoods, I became more familiar with what poverty and racism had done to the African American people who lived there. I was appalled. Clearly, they had been screwed by the same system from which I had benefited.

The first summer, I worked for a neonatologist at Evanston Hospital. My pediatrician, Herbert Philipsborn, had set me up on the job. He had gone to school with my father and was a family friend. He knew I was interested in science – particularly biochemistry. He thought an experience in a hospital might stimulate an interest in medicine. I lived at home and went to work each day on the Northwestern railroad. My job was to count the vessels in the umbilical cords of all babies born at the hospital and photograph the ears of all newborn babies. Umbilical cords normally have one vein and two arteries. Occasionally one had just a vein and one artery. It turned out these babies were more likely to have other abnormalities. I photographed the babies' ears to see whether these pictures were just as good as fingerprints or footprints. These were easy, mindless jobs and I got to go on rounds with the doctor and see how a medical service ran.

One day, I was asked to go to the morgue to see the autopsy of one of the babies with abnormal umbilical vessels and to infuse the placenta with dyes. Predictably, the morgue was in the bowels of the hospital. I remembered how I had fainted in high school, and I was very apprehensive about what would happen. I braced myself and opened the door. I was hit by the smell of formaldehyde mixed with a stench I later learned was that of human internal organs. (The same smell accompanies operations on living humans.) The first thing I saw was a nude male corpse on a stainless-steel table. Next to that was another stainless-steel table with a gray/white infant corpse and a placenta next to it. The pathologist was dressed in a hospital gown and scrubs, and he turned and welcomed me with a big smile.

"So! You want to see an autopsy and examine the vessels of the placenta?" He was enthusiastic about his work, but he was pale, wilted and pasty as if he spent his life underground in purgatory. Nevertheless, in a morose way, I wanted to see the dissection of the human body. I had never seen a dead body before. I was just a naive 18-year-old who had never seen a naked man.

The man on the table looked about 60 and he had thinning gray hair and coarse features. He was slightly overweight. His body was a grayish blue especially near the steel bench – he was pinker on the top. His penis was retracted, and his scrotum was darkish blue. I tried to distance myself from this person – but thoughts of his family, his job, his personality snuck into my mind. If I thought too much about the personal issues, I felt somewhat panicked. I had to repress these thoughts. It's just a body. Dead. It has to be examined to learn information that will help other people in the future. As long as I thought about these last things, I was okay.

The pathologist began with the head. He cut through the scalp from ear to ear across the top of the head as if tracing the line of headphones over the dome. He then cut and pulled the skin back to the neck and forward over the face (crumpling the identity of the person) and exposed the entire skull. Next, he brought out an electric saw and cut a circle along a track as if it was the band of a baseball cap. Then using a regular hammer and a chisel, he popped the top off. There was a membrane and underneath it the brain: a pale cream color with delicate curves and interspersed blue and maroon vessels. Unfixed, it had the quality of a pristine, almost translucent vanilla custard. The pathologist "delivered" the brain, weighed it on a scale and delicately placed it in a jar of formaldehyde to fix it for microscopic examination. He then went on to open the abdomen and chest to remove the other organs. These organs inside smelled! They were also coarse and bloody. I was surprised how thick the skin and subcutaneous tissue was – how much fat there is in the abdomen. In contrast, the brain seemed delicate, clean and pure.

Next, the pathologist proceeded to the child. This was surprisingly easier than the man because the baby was clearly grossly deformed with organs protruding from its abdomen. The baby's face was deformed – compressed probably from the delivery. It had died within hours of birth. The pathologist showed me how he could perfuse the arteries of the placenta with red dye and the veins with green dye and then put the organ in a clearing solution that made the substance of the organ translucent. The vessels could be seen in detail. Although these preparations were beautiful, I'm not sure what new knowledge we gained from them.

Back at school, despite going out to bars and smoking dope, I was getting very good grades. I was a chemistry major and philosophy and art history minor. There were only nine chemistry majors in my year, which meant I had the run of the labs and could work on independent projects whenever I wanted. I didn't take an English course because it required reading a book a week and that was a total impossibility for me.

I survived academically because I was a morning person. We all went out and got trashed in the late evening (Figure 2.1), but

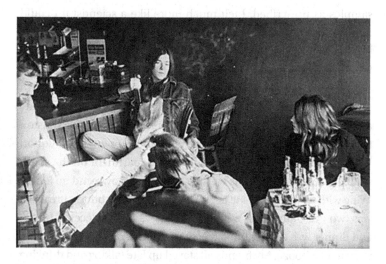

Figure 2.1 Me in bar with friends. Courtesy of Vassar College.

I came back to the dorm by midnight, woke up the next morning, ate breakfast and went to all my classes no matter how I felt. I didn't have an alarm clock. I just woke up early. I relied on my notes for the tests, and I had an organized plan for studying for exams. All my friends were English or Art History majors, but I wanted to be a scientist or maybe a scientist doctor. Ultimately, two of the pigs became addicted to heroin, one was murdered in Washington, DC and one was kicked out the day before graduation. Three others graduated as expected.

The next summer working at a hospital, I was allowed to focus on more biochemical work, running electrophoretic gels on haptoglobin samples of each of the newborns. During these summer jobs, I was expected to analyze various proteins in blood using standard laboratory equipment. I looked to improve the efficiency of the methods and double or triple the number of samples I could run each day. Instead of just running the samples as prescribed, I felt much more like a scientist if I could improve the experiments.

This second summer, I lived with Les Moore and a couple of friends down in Hyde Park near the University of Chicago. I was determined to make it on my own. I was paid only $200 a month and so to make ends meet I had to budget carefully. I had to pay a share of the rent, buy my ticket on the train to get to Evanston Hospital (on the other side of the city) and buy food and liquor. It took an hour and a half to get from our apartment on the south side to Evanston, but it was worth it to be on my own and no longer living with my parents. I ate eggs, bread and peanut butter. Breakfast was two eggs; lunch was a hardboiled egg and two pieces of bread; and dinner was two scrambled eggs with toast. Any money left over went to buy booze. My friends all stayed up late talking and drinking and I went to bed early so I could go to work the next day. On the Elevated Rail Line (the El), everyone stood away from me because I wore a lab coat splattered with blood.

Dr. Philipsborn suggested I apply to institutions offering a combined MD/PhD program. If I got both degrees, I could work in the lab and/or with patients. So, I decided to apply to both PhD and MD/PhD programs. To do that, I had to take the MCAT exams (the standardized entrance exams for medical school). Unfortunately, the date of the exam was May 1. Derby Day.

At school, I had a friend from Louisville whose father worked for a bank and had box tickets to the Kentucky Derby. She invited me. I said I couldn't go because the MCAT exam was the same day. Take them in Louisville! I signed up and matched to Louisville.

We drove all night and arrived at her house in Louisville on Friday morning. A maid greeted us with two big mint juleps in silver cups that we guzzled down and we then went to sleep. That afternoon, we went to the Oaks – an afternoon of filly races. We made small bets on some of the races, but I didn't win anything.

Saturday morning, I put on a sleeveless dress for the Derby and went off to the university to take the test. The women registering students told me that I couldn't possibly be taking the MCATs and corrected me – I must be taking the SATs to get into college. When I told her I was sure I'd signed up for the MCATs, she insisted that I was wrong. Finally, after several more back-and-forths, I was allowed to take the right test. I was the only girl in the room, and I took a seat in the corner.

The proctor had her hair in a pink beehive hairdo and wore five-inch heels and a tight pink dress. She admonished all of us not to use notes, not to talk to each other and not to leave the room. As soon as the test began, she left the room. Immediately, all the guys started talking to each other, pulling out notes and leaving the room. The periodic chart of the elements was on the wall. Was I at a disadvantage?

When the test was over, the proctor was picked up outside by a guy in a pink Cadillac who was obviously destined for the Derby. I went too, of course, and what a phenomenon it was. Women in their huge hats and spring dresses, men with stogies buying $1,000 tickets on the horses and hawkers selling mint juleps in the stands (Figure 2.2). We had a great time, but my test scores were miserable. I expected low scores as my dyslexia meant I always failed to finish many sections. Despite my low scores, I got interviews at Rockefeller University for the PhD but didn't get in – those "R" schools (Radcliffe and Rockefeller) were jinxed. I got interviews at Johns Hopkins and the University of Wisconsin for the MD/PhD program. Wisconsin had a federally funded MD/PhD program whereas Hopkins said they had one "you design yourself."

In November, one of my chemistry professors asked me to come to tea after dinner to meet an alumna, Dr. Mary Betty Stevens, who was a professor at Hopkins. My professor warned me to behave myself and wear a skirt. I guess my training for the debutante ball

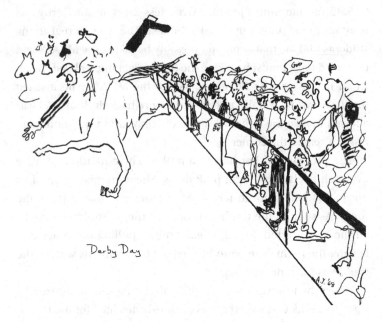

Derby Day

A.Y.68

Figure 2.2 Derby Day, 1968.

was useful because I did what she told me and within a few weeks I was accepted early admission to Hopkins.

During my senior year, I worked with Professor Anne Gounaris who had received her PhD from Radcliffe and then worked with the famous enzyme biochemist, Daniel E. Koshland. Her large biochemistry laboratory was at my disposal. Lab work was fun because I was in control. I could design my own experiments, carry them out and get the results. I was assigned a project to purify and characterize yeast pyruvate decarboxylase. This enzyme is important in the formation of alcohol (ethanol) during fermentation. The enzyme was likely regulated by vitamin B1 and other factors because it was in a terminal part of the Krebs cycle – a key cycle in energy metabolism. Purifying the enzyme would

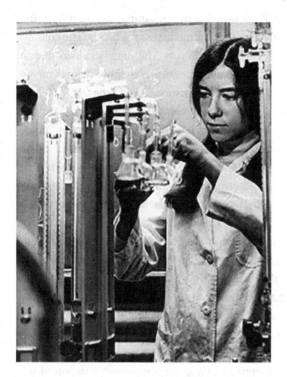

Figure 2.3 Me examining sample on the Warburg apparatus. Courtesy of Vassar College.

reveal how it is regulated in the cell and teach me methods of protein purification and characterization.

The usual way to measure this enzyme's activity was to use something called the Warburg apparatus. Unfortunately, it could only measure activity in 12 samples in several hours (Figure 2.3). I was trying to purify the enzyme with gel chromatography. Chromatography in this case involved putting an enzyme solution on top of a two-foot-tall glass column filled with special beads, pouring a buffer on top after the sample and collecting 2 milliliter (about 1 teaspoon) samples as the liquid comes out the bottom of the column. The various proteins in the sample separate from the others as they travel down the column across the beads. The column generated dozens of samples each run. The drawback was that to evaluate the purification, I had to measure enzyme activity in all the many samples, but I could only measure 12 at a time.

Consequently, I spent many weekend mornings in the chemistry library, looking for possible simple colorimetric assays to measure crude pyruvate decarboxylase activity rapidly. I modified some older methods that used dyes to interact specifically with an aldehyde that was an intermediate in the pyruvate decarboxylase reaction. I could use just a few drops of each fraction coming off the chromatographic column to measure activity in minutes. Thus, I could combine enzyme-rich fractions quickly and purify them further. I could carry out experiments to characterize the kinetics and regulation of the enzyme.

I found that phenylalanine had profound effects on the enzyme by allosterically altering the reactions. Allosteric reactions occur in biology when a molecule interacts on a specific site on its appointed protein and then a second molecule acts on a separate site on the same protein thereby changing the shape and function of the original protein. The papers originally describing allosteric reactions by Monod, Wyman and Changeux were published in 1965, my freshman year. The allosteric properties were further defined by Koshland, Nemethy, and Filmer in 1966. I was instantly fascinated by this kind of control of biochemical reactions in our bodies. Such allosteric control of protein shape and function later proved the basis of many drug actions and unique 'infections' based on protein shape-changing – the prion diseases such as mad cow disease and Creutzfeldt–Jakob disease.

I wrote my honors thesis based on these observations. The morning of my oral defense I woke up with terrible laryngitis and could only croak out words. I prepared myself a thermos of tea and honey and did my best, sipping intermittently on the soothing liquid. As was not unusual for me, I was very animated and almost hypomanic in my presentation. I remember my organic chemistry teacher interrupting to ask what I had in the thermos. When it comes to presenting in front of an audience, I have always felt very nervous but also confident about my knowledge of a topic.

I graduated summa cum laude in chemistry and thirteenth in the 1969 class of 400. When I went to get in line with the top 20 students, the two students on either side of me asked me why I was there. I said I had been instructed to stand there. They said they didn't even know I went to Vassar. They thought I was a townie. I had made a hydroxyhexane molecule out of a chemistry model kit. It was a ring with a little side chain like a tassel. I hid it under the sleeve of my gown, and when I went up to get my degree I whipped off my cap and put on my molecule. A real chemistry major!

The summer before medical school, I basically lounged around. I spent time on the farm, and back in Winnetka I got all my things together for school. During the summer, I had several bad stomach aches that my pediatrician couldn't understand. He recommended that I have my appendix out since after all who needs an appendix anyway and it could be the cause of my stomach aches. I was alright with that.

I was admitted electively and had general anesthesia. The surgeons made a long vertical incision because once inside my abdomen, they decided to take a good look around. The appendix was apparently mildly inflamed but everything else was alright. My mother was sitting by the side of my bed when I came to from the anesthesia. I was curled up on my side. As I woke up and rolled over, I found I was lying in a large pool of blood. My IV had become disconnected from the needle, and I had managed to gradually bleed out slowly for about an hour. My first inpatient hospital experience. It would not be my last.

3
• • • • •

One of 10 Women
in a Class of 114

I met Jack, officially known as John Bradbury Penney, Jr., at the reception at Dean David Roger's house the night before my first day at Johns Hopkins School of Medicine (Figure 3.1). Most of the students were dressed up and looking very straight. I joined a bunch of people hovering together who had more facial hair and seemed more liberal. Jack was one of them and he was expounding on being a member of Students for a Democratic Society (SDS) and how awful the Vietnam War was. I mostly agreed with his opinions, although I wasn't in favor of the violence groups like SDS espoused. I also found him way too vocal and aggressive. I didn't realize it at the time, but a loud and talkative Jack was a break from his usual quiet personality. We all went out after the reception to drink beer. I was thinking that this medical school thing might be a drag. I couldn't see myself hanging out with the guys wearing ties and jackets, but I wasn't exactly charmed by the loudmouth liberals with whom I presumably had more in common.

The first weekend I was in Baltimore, there was a party at the Pithotomy Club, an eating club for male medical students

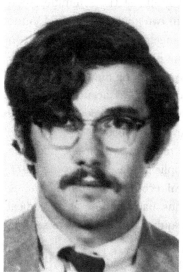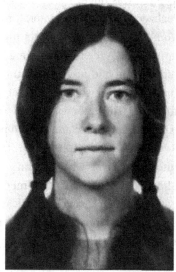

Figure 3.1 John (Jack) Bradbury Penney, Jr. and Anne Buckingham Young.

only. Female medical students and nurses were invited to parties, and I decided to go. The party was a typical medical student party with lots of beer and dancing. All of a sudden, we heard shots ring out on the street. The medical students rushed out onto the street. A man had been shot right in front of the club. A real opportunity for the students to practice their skills! They crowded over him, trying to revive him by CPR and attempting to stop the bleeding from the wound. A group of them carried him up the street to the emergency room.

A month or two after starting medical school, a biochemistry graduate student asked me to go with him to his professor's house for a party. At the door I was introduced to the professor. "Anne Young! Oh, I have a great story to tell you!" He said he was on the Admissions Committee when my application came up for review.

The file was huge. Twice the size of others! The committee soon realized it contained material from two applicants named 'Anne Young.' They spent an entire meeting sorting out the two applicants. After finally getting one pile of the Anne Young they didn't want and a second of the Anne Young they did want, they had to contend with a letter that couldn't be associated with one or the other. The letter was from a psychiatrist who said, "Anne Young is completely crazy and should never be a doctor."

I didn't say anything. I wanted to get away from the door and into the party. *I* was the crazy applicant described in the letter. I had naively allowed *all* my medical records to be submitted along with my medical school applications. Back in those days, medical schools encouraged (but didn't require) the applicant to send in records.

I stood there while the host professor told me that Hopkins Professor Mary Betty Stevens (a Vassar alumna) had checked me out at Vassar and decided that I was fine. I took a deep breath. I had gotten into med school by the seat of my pants.

My first impressions of the people I'd gravitated to that first night at the dean's house gradually became more positive as I got to know and become part of a small group of students who sat at the back of the lecture hall, reading the *New York Times* and talking about civil rights, the antiwar movement, drugs and the need to help the poor. I learned quickly that Jack was a very quiet man – not the loudmouth I saw the first night. He also had an incredible fund of knowledge having read the entire *Encyclopedia Britannica* when he was a child. Our group became lifelong friends and colleagues: Walter Henze, Darrell Salk (son of Jonas Salk who produced the first polio vaccine), Jack, Jeremy Tuttle and me.

Whenever Jack sat near me, I noticed this really bad smell coming from under the chairs. I soon realized that the smell emanated from Jack's feet. In his attempts to be a hippie, he wore jeans, wool shirts and Birkenstocks with no socks. His feet sweat and his sandals stank.

In my usual subtle way, I said that if he didn't fix the stink in his feet, he shouldn't sit next to me. He did fix it! He started wearing socks (and as I learned later, he was spraying his feet with foot powder). He got a new pair of Birkenstocks. That was my first sign that he liked me. And I liked him.

A group of us attended the big Second Anti-War Moratorium in Washington, DC on November 15, 1969, to protest the senseless Vietnam War in which too many Americans were dying. Although we weren't exactly invited to help, we decided to go and be prepared to help any people who were hurt or fell ill. The war felt very real to us especially because Jack had received a very low lottery number from the Draft Board – meaning if he wasn't in medical school, he would have been drafted into military service. We wore our white coats and black armbands and were prepared to take care of minor wounds and tear gas with water bottles and cloth strips. There were half a million protesters and by the end of the evening the march deteriorated into throwing sticks and stones. The police heavily tear-gassed the crowd. At least we had water-soaked pieces of cloth to help people breathe and see.

That spring, Jack announced that on March 7 there was going to be a total eclipse of the sun. He always followed celestial events by reading the relevant sections of the *Baltimore Sun* and *Scientific American*. The band of totality was going to fall across the southern tip of the Eastern Shore of Maryland and northern Virginia. Walter, Jack, Lynne Gerson (a fellow medical student) and I decided to miss classes to go and see it, since this was the event of a lifetime. We got in Walter's VW and started off toward the Eastern Shore. It was spring and the weather was clear and fresh. We had to go over the 4-mile-long Chesapeake Bay Bridge to the Eastern Shore and I thanked my lucky stars I wasn't driving. We drove on as far as we could until we were way down the shore and out in the boonies with no clear idea of where we were. At about 10 p.m., we came to a dirt road and followed it until we found a little place where we could put down our sleeping bags. We all fell asleep. It was chilly but we were all excited about the next day.

As the first light came, there were sudden explosions all around us! What was happening? It was gunfire! We were petrified when we realized that we were on the edge of some marshes and guns were being fired from several directions. We were in the middle of a duck-hunting preserve! We instantly packed up our sleeping bags and stuffed them in the car and hightailed it out of there. We got back on a paved road and decided to try to get as far south as possible. When we neared the end of the peninsula, there were stretches of salt marshes. We parked and picked a path out into the marshes. It was an absolutely clear, cool, cloudless day. We pulled out a joint and got stoned. Rushes lined the pathway, and you could see up and out but couldn't see anything beyond five feet side to side. We walked out along the path and, after about half a mile, we turned a corner and there in front of us was a clear area where a man and his young son had set up all sorts of equipment to see the eclipse. He had several telescopes and cameras on tripods. He had a large white sheet spread out and anchored by rocks to see the interference waves in the seconds before totality. The guy was very nice and invited us to stay. He was obviously an astronomy buff and Jack was absolutely thrilled.

As the eclipse began, we looked at it through the man's special telescope and pinhole projections on the ground. As totality neared, we noted that all the shadows became absolutely crisp since the sun was closer to a point source. When I held out my hair, I could distinguish all the individual hairs! As it got darker, it got colder by about 15 degrees. The shore birds started returning to land en masse somewhat confused about what was going on. As totality approached, interference bands raced across the spread-out sheet and suddenly the sun winked out and all we could see was a ring of fire surrounding the moon. It lasted several minutes, and we all relished the moment together in this most beautiful of places. After the event, we piled back in the VW and headed back to school feeling a little richer for the shared experience. Along the way, we stopped to eat, and Walter ate three dozen raw oysters in celebration. That night, he became terribly ill to his stomach as a consequence of his gluttony.

That trip was the longest time I had spent with Jack. I liked him.

That spring, Jack and I spent more and more time together. In May, I invited him and Walter Henze to my room to watch the Kentucky Derby, drink mint juleps and bet on the races. When I was young my mother liked to say, "Why don't you call up one of your friends to play." I was sure they would hate it if I called. I was always hoping someone might call *me* up to come over. Even as an adult, I avoided calling strangers on the phone and had to work up my courage to call Jack and Walter, who accepted my invitation. When the day came, I set up the mint juleps and had snacks and the TV all ready. But they didn't show up. I was crushed. Later, I found out they'd decided to go out with someone else. In the end, it didn't really matter because two weeks later we all went to the Preakness Stakes in Baltimore and watched the horses from the infield. Three years later, we saw Secretariat win the Preakness as part of winning the Triple Crown – winning the Kentucky Derby, the Preakness Stakes and the Belmont Stakes.

Plenty of the medical school lectures at Johns Hopkins were dry and boring, but some lecturers were remarkable. Professor Richard T. Johnson, a neurologist who pioneered studies of viruses infecting the nervous system, showed exciting movies of his research trips in the field. He showed an unforgettable film of a remote tribe in the mountains of Papua New Guinea that suffered a strikingly tragic and fatal disease called kuru. The disease caused trembling, followed by shrinkage and wasting of the muscles and loss of all coordination, resulting in death in one to two years. In 1964, Johnson joined the medical researcher D. Carleton Gajdusek in Papua New Guinea and filmed people affected by kuru. His movies showed the amazingly disorderly movements of the affected individuals. Gajdusek had demonstrated that people contracted the disease via their funerary rite of smearing the brains of dead relatives on their bodies. Whether it was a virus, bacteria, parasite or something else was unknown. Jack and I met Gajdusek at Johnson's house one evening where he talked about his adventures and his theories of what caused kuru. We decided then that it would be cool to be part of a study that took us to remote parts of the world – a wish that came true years later when we did field research in Venezuelan stilt villages.

Whereas Johnson kept his lectures interesting with exciting medical content, more typically professors resorted to what was apparently an approved gimmick to keep the students' attention: sprinkle every lecture with slides of *Playboy* pinups or lewd jokes. There were only 10 women in our class of 114 and so the women were expected to just tolerate the lewd material. I noticed that Jack and his 'liberal' friends were just as sexist as the rest of the class. Once when a woman gave an incredibly lucid lecture on infectious disease, all the guys tuned out almost as a matter of principle. It really pissed me off and I told Jack that I felt that way. He admitted that he'd tuned out and was embarrassed about it.

Despite this crude educational approach, there were two women at Hopkins who really impressed me. One was Professor Helen Taussig, a pediatric cardiologist who went completely deaf as she got older and thus couldn't use a stethoscope to listen for various kinds of murmurs. Nevertheless, she could diagnose the most complex child by simple observation and the feel of the vibrations in the chest. Truly extraordinary. The other woman was Chief Resident in Medicine – a position reserved for the best – who had graduated from Vassar several years ahead of me and then attended Harvard Medical School. I once saw her present a complicated patient at Grand Rounds before a large audience and a front row seated with the giants of Hopkins Medicine – A. McGehee Harvey, Philip Tumulty and Victor McKusick. She was blonde, and in a short white skirt and short white jacket, she reminded me of Barbie, the doll. She spoke for 15 minutes summarizing all the details of the patient without pause and without uttering a single 'Um' or 'Ah.' It was perfect. She then confidently answered all the intentionally tough questions posed by the greats – again in full sentences without pauses. Bernadine Healy later became the first female director of the National Institutes of Health. These two women taught me to maintain confidence, never quit and to continue on despite barriers.

Summer was fast approaching. I wanted to work in a lab. Who should I work with? There were so many possibilities.

I asked multiple graduate students in different departments who I should talk to. Several people who knew of my potential interest in the brain suggested I speak with Solomon Snyder. He was then a young man who had recently joined the faculty of the pharmacology department while at the same time finishing his residency in psychiatry. He was working on neurotransmitters and drug effects on the brain.

I made an appointment to see him and was so excited that I went to the library and put together a proposal to study the effects of the blood pressure drug reserpine on potential amino acid neurotransmitters. Sol had lectured on reserpine and its effects on adrenaline release. Maybe it had an effect on other potential neurotransmitters.

Sol's office was on the fifth floor of one of the main medical school buildings a block from the hospital. The office door opened into a room where his secretary was working at a desk next to another door to his office.

I announced myself and his secretary knocked on the door. Sol came out to meet me. He was thin, about 5'10" and had light brown hair. I'm not sure what kind of person I expected but I immediately felt at ease. He did not appear physically strong, and his handshake was surprisingly weak. With a soft voice, he motioned me into his office. A large window looked out over the poor neighborhood below. His desk faced away from the window toward the inside of the office. There was a sitting area with a couch backed up against the desk and two chairs facing the couch. A whiteboard on the wall had lots of scribbles on it. I took a seat in one of the chairs.

"What can I help you with?" he asked.

"Well, I'm really interested in the brain and biochemistry. I'd like to learn more about it. I actually wrote a proposal for a lab project for the summer." I handed him a copy of my proposal.

He looked it over politely as we talked. He asked me about my previous lab work, and I told him about my summers working in hospitals and my college honors thesis. I found him easy and enjoyable to interact with. He was so supportive and enthusiastic about my exploring brain chemistry that I came right out and asked, "Would it be possible to join your lab this summer?"

He did not hesitate. "Absolutely. I can provide you with a small stipend as well."

What great news. Now I had this exciting summer of science ahead.

Most of the medical students lived in a dormitory across the street from the hospital. There was a basketball court and a swimming pool by the building. One evening, Jack and I sat by the pool talking and a second-year medical student came up, looked down at me and said, "Women shouldn't be doctors. They should be at home taking care of the children and their husbands!" My playground instincts instantly returned. I jumped up, looked him in the eye, hauled off and hit him as hard as I could right between the eyes. He didn't fall back much at all and instead he hauled off and hit me back, decking me to the ground. Jack didn't do anything in response but just let it all play out. Clearly the wisest response.

I moved out of the medical school dorm at the end of my first year when two college friends, both taking creative writing courses at Hopkins, moved out of their apartment at 311 East 30th Street near the main Hopkins campus a couple of miles from the medical school. I moved into the apartment with Les Moore, who'd begun a job working in a sleep physiology laboratory in Baltimore. She brought along her boyfriend. As far as I could tell, he was neither going to school nor working. When I came home from work, Les and I and the boyfriend got stoned and/or drunk and hung out.

I was 22 that summer and it was my first time working in a pharmacology lab. That year, 1970, was the year the Nobel Prize in Physiology or Medicine went to three scientists for discovering how chemical transmission worked between a nerve cell and the next neuron, gland or organ. At the time, physiologists specialized in recording brain electrical activity in response to specific behaviors. Although most thought that chemical transmission between nerve cells did exist, the prevailing belief was that transmission was primarily electrical. Electrical activity could be measured in living animals and was still considered to be a factor, but the Nobel work was groundbreaking in that it showcased the important role played by chemical transmission.

Sol Snyder had been a student of Julius Axelrod, a member of the Nobel Prize–winning team. So, by the time Sol came to Hopkins, he had already been intimately involved in the research that led to the discovery of the first chemical transmitters. His lab was to continue research into the chemistry of the brain. When I began my lab work, only four chemicals were widely considered as neurotransmitters: acetylcholine, dopamine, norepinephrine and GABA (gamma-aminobutyric acid). We had no clue at the time about the chemical transmitters for 90 percent of the brain neurons.

Neurotransmitters are basically messengers in the brain. They are chemicals released by nerve cell activation. The junction between one nerve cell and the next is called a synapse (Figure 3.2). Small vesicles (beads of membrane filled with the transmitter) fuse with

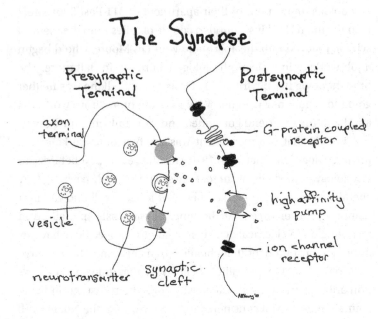

The Synapse

Presynaptic Terminal

Postsynaptic Terminal

axon terminal

G-protein coupled receptor

vesicle

high affinity pump

neurotransmitter

synaptic cleft

ion channel receptor

Figure 3.2 The synapse.

There are trillions of synapses in the human brain. Each synapse is unique but influenced by the other neighboring synapses. The transmitter is stored in vesicles that fuse with the presynaptic membrane to release the messenger when the presynaptic terminal is activated. The transmitter diffuses across the synaptic cleft to activate specific postsynaptic receptors. The transmitter action is then terminated by special potent pumps that remove the transmitter from the cleft.

the surface of the nerve ending at the synapse. The transmitter is released into the synaptic cleft and diffuses across to the next nerve cell where it binds to a receptor like a key in a lock. This is how the signal is passed on. Of course, as in a well-tuned security system, the receptors are very specific and selective and will only interact with certain chemicals. At each step, the processes in the brain can be modified by various enzymes, proteins, vitamins, hormones and drugs. The four accepted neurotransmitters we knew about thus far were all unique chemicals not used in any of the body's other cellular functions.

60

In Sol's lab, several postdoctoral fellows were looking at amino acids as potential neurotransmitters. We knew that amino acids are the basic building blocks of proteins that are found in every cell in the body. Could they also be involved in something completely different than building proteins? If so, how could amino acids both be critical components of proteins and have secondary functions as neurotransmitters? There are 20 amino acids and each is present in high concentrations in all body parts. Could any or all of those 20 be involved in neurotransmission? Even the question was controversial back then. Identifying any of them as a neurotransmitter would open up opportunities to find drugs that affect their functioning. Finding new transmitters of any kind would allow scientists to develop a more complete map of the brain's neurotransmitter pathways. For all these reasons, I was excited to be involved in the study of amino acids as potential neurotransmitters. It was then a significant, cutting-edge area of research where discoveries could be made.

Over the summer, Jack went back to his home in Boston to work in a lab at the University of Massachusetts. Between the time he stood me up for the Kentucky Derby and the end of the term, we'd made love in my little dormitory room and fallen in love. I adored his sparkly hazel eyes, his thick beard and hairy chest. He had a strong body. He smelled good. He was quiet yet always knew the right information. We both wanted to be together, and I knew I would miss him when he was in Boston. Jack and I wrote letters back and forth and his were very cute and clever. I don't think he saved my letters – if he did, I don't know where they are. We managed to get together a couple of times over the summer.

One long weekend, Walter and I visited Jack at his grandmother's farm in southern New Hampshire. We arrived around five in the afternoon and Jack's father came out to greet us. "Hi," he said cheerfully. That's the last word I heard from him all weekend. Jack's mom and grandmothers were talkative and interactive. Meanwhile

Jack's dad smiled and laughed and served the food and helped with the dishes but didn't say anything to any of us. I asked Jack what was going on and he said that his dad was just a bit shy and a man of few words.

During the week, work in Sol's lab kept me busy. Sol had put me on a project measuring the level of histamine (a chemical associated with allergies) in the rat brain. A prior member of his lab had found high levels in the brain. What was it doing there? Could it be a neurotransmitter? First, I measured the localization of the histamine in the nerve cells. I then measured the histamine at various ages of the rat. I found out that the increased histamine was greatest in the newborn brain. It was highest in the nucleus of the cell and very low in the synaptic terminal where neurotransmission took place. My experiments allowed us to rule out histamine as a neurotransmitter – more likely involved in the development of the brain and the function of the nucleus.

Five or six postdoctoral fellows and several students shared the lab with me that summer, and by the time I got to work at 8 a.m. somebody else was already there. Each of us had an assigned work area at one of the six lab benches. We all had different backgrounds and training, which made our frequent scientific and political discussions especially interesting. We might argue loudly and vehemently, but no one was aggressive. Sol was brilliant and fun to talk to about science.

Sol's lab was right next to his office, which made it easy for him to meet weekly with each lab member. He carefully went over all the actual numbers in my lab book, looking for any additional information in the data I might have missed. If experiments were outside his expertise, he didn't hesitate to call up a colleague and arrange for me to go learn a new technique in the colleague's laboratory. I was excited by the work in the lab and was eager to be someone who made discoveries in the world. Discovering more about transmitters and drugs in the brain was definitely an adventure. During college, when I'd sat around with my English major friends who talked about books, I wasn't a match because my dyslexia meant I was very ignorant of classic literature. Instead, I was the scientist among the Pigs. I'd say, *someday we're gonna be able to manipulate the genetics of our systems. We might be able to cure diseases or create monsters.* I liked to think about all the things humans might come up with.

Sol was willing to listen to my ideas and guided me in how to examine them. Julius Axelrod had taught him to design short 'pilot' experiments to test out new ideas. Some scientists are inclined to carry out long, large, all-inclusive experiments right out of the starting gate. Such experiments often failed not because of the design but rather because the experiments were too large and unwieldy. Better to design a shorter and smaller 12-tube experiment that indicated 'yes' or 'no' about the central idea.

During another long weekend visiting Jack in New Hampshire, he took me for a walk out across the field by a ledge and down the slope to where a grove of small beech trees crossed the field. A path wound its way through the cluster of thin trunks and then broke away into another little meadow that stretched up a slope. The meadow was covered with the most delightful speckling of little red dots – wild strawberries. We spent hours picking until we had about two quarts of the precious, tiny berries. Jack's mother, who put up all sorts of fruits every year, helped us decide how to preserve the berries. We decided that it might be fun to try the recipe for 'sunshine strawberries' from Fannie Farmer's cookbook. We mixed the berries with sugar, boiled them for 20 minutes and then spread them on glass platters and covered them with plastic wrap. We put them on the roof of the house in the full sun. The next day we both had to go back to school, so we put them on the shelf above the rear seat in Piglet, my VW bug, and tootled back to Baltimore where we put them on the roof again for three more days and then packed them up into sterilized glass jars and sealed them with wax. I don't think Jack and I have ever tasted better strawberry preserves.

I loved to visit the farm in New Hampshire. Jack's mom was always making something delicious. She taught me how to make several breads that Jack and I then made routinely back in Baltimore. She made an excellent roast and then whipped up Yorkshire pudding with the grease. Her soups and stews were outstanding, and we always had frozen fresh vegetables grown in her garden. She and I had several other projects together such as stenciling a border of flowers around one of the upstairs bedrooms in the farmhouse. She was so easy to talk to and we talked about all sorts of practical and funny things. Although she didn't approve of sugar in tea, which meant I quickly learned to drink tea 'neat,' she was unlike my mother, who was always critical and argumentative. From the beginning, I was always completely comfortable with Margaret.

Jack and I loved to swim and often the weather at the farm became hot and oppressive. When it did, we drove the quick five-minute ride down to the dam on Bow Lake and went for a delicious swim in the fresh, clean water. The lake was beautiful with little islands sprinkled around the periphery and a dam at one end which controlled the water level. It is a glacial lake and there was no public access, so we had to have a little medallion to prove we had a right to swim there. The only problem with the lake was that once we had gone for a swim and were refreshed, we had to dry off, get in the car and head back to the farm. By the end of the short five-minute drive, we were hot and sweaty again.

At the end of the summer rotation, I asked Sol if I could get my PhD in his laboratory in the Department of Pharmacology. I had a year and a half left of my science and clinical rotations and I proposed joining the lab after that. He said there should be no problem. I made an appointment to meet with the dean. At the time, the Hopkins MD program had only 2.5 years of required courses.

The rest were elective. I asked the dean if I could use all my elective time toward getting my PhD. He agreed. I asked if he would put that in writing. He gave me such a letter the next week.

I then went to the pharmacology department and asked the chair if I could get a PhD in their department working in Sol's lab and he said yes.

"Could the Medical School courses in biochemistry, physiology and pharmacology count for the PhD?" I asked. This seemed reasonable since various departments counted these courses for graduate students.

"Yes," they said again.

I asked if I could get that in writing and they gave me a letter soon thereafter. I must say I don't know what drove me to ask for those letters, but it turned out to be a good thing later.

4

• • • • •

Surviving the Courses and Clinical Rotations

In the fall, Jack and Walter moved into an apartment on Washington Square. Jack began spending more and more time in my apartment, sleeping with me in my single bed. Gradually, he brought over his clothes and his books. We hung out and maybe played squash or went hiking together. It was more fun being with him than without him. Besides, he knew everything. He'd read the pharmacology, microbiology and pathology textbooks in no time flat while I was struggling to read 10–20 pages per night. I discovered that I could kind of look at the overall gist of the chapters we were supposed to be studying and then I could pick Jack's brain about what was actually in them. He was a master at summarizing all the key stuff while avoiding all the irrelevant details. Like his dad, he was a man of few words, but he could distill huge amounts of information to an essence. I found that as long as I went to class to hear the lectures and discussed issues with Jack, I could essentially pass medical school courses without reading any textbooks. I read little sections of chapters to the extent that I had time. If Jack hadn't been with me, I don't know how I would have learned the material. I read too slowly and didn't retain it well either. The beauty of being with Jack was that I learned so much from him and it was much more fun than learning alone.

In the second year of medical school, we had a neuroscience course. One morning, the professor introduced a person who had Parkinson's disease. A stooped man about 60 years old walked in with short stiff steps and had difficulty walking up the four steps to the stage of the lecture hall. His speech was almost inaudible. The use of his hands was limited but he had no shaking (tremor). After this brief encounter, the professor gave the man a pill of L-Dopa – a brand-new therapy for Parkinson's disease – and then asked the man to sit down while he finished his lecture. After the cause and symptoms of Parkinson's disease were presented, the professor called the man back up on stage. The man stood up quickly and nimbly and trotted up to the stage! It was a miracle I'll never forget. This tiny pill had reversed his symptoms. The pill was replenishing a supply of one neurotransmitter – dopamine! If this could be done for Parkinson's, could it be done for other diseases? This lecture had a major influence on my career choice. Jack was amazed by it as well. The fact that Parkinson's could be diagnosed simply by observing the person's problems with motor agility, posture, balance and finger dexterity was so appealing. No need for blood tests. At the time, brain scans were not available but brand-new effective therapies were.

We all had to take a course on the chest x-ray, which met once a week at 1 p.m. As usual, the professor periodically showed pictures of nude women. When I noticed that the professor put his slides in the slide projector's carousel and then left for lunch, I concocted a plan and contacted a friend in pathology. The pathology residents were the only ones who could easily get a color slide made because they had the photographic setup for making slides of various pathologic human organs. My friend went down to the 'Block' in Baltimore – the red-light district – bought a magazine with a picture of a guy in full-frontal nudity standing on a cliff, his muscular body all greased up and a big dick hanging down, and made it into a slide. During lunch, when the professor was out, I slipped the slide into his carousel.

About midway through class, when my slide of the nude male came up, the professor became instantly pale. He clicked rapidly to the next slide – a regular chest x-ray. The guys in the class, however, all said, "Whoaaaa. Back it up. The girls want to see this." He had to reverse the slides. He was confused; maybe the slide was his? Eventually, this professor found out that the nude male was my slide, but he never showed a *Playboy* pinup in class again. I suffered no ramifications.

Going forward, there were fewer slides of nude females in any lectures. As I continued to do throughout my life, I had taken the Pippi Longstocking approach, which I defined as approaching problems and interpersonal conflicts from a mischievous angle. Rather than coming on strong and serious, why not use a sense of humor?

Sometime in the late fall, Les Moore's boyfriend walked out, and Les decided that sleep physiology wasn't for her and that she was going to go out to Oregon to live with her older sister, Lucy, on a lesbian commune. I told her this seemed to be a poor way to get over her relationship with this worthless boyfriend let alone a way of starting a new career. She didn't listen, however, and off she went leaving Jack and me missing her.

We (or rather I) had to find a new roommate to share the rent as Jack was sharing rent with Walter. I met with women medical students at one of the monthly lunches. There were only 9 or 10 women in each class of 110. One of the women in the class below me, Nancy Serrell, wanted to get out of the dorm and without having even seen the apartment volunteered to be my roommate. Little did she know what she was getting into. She was a bit shy but fun to be with and she brought along tons of Joni Mitchell and Phoebe Snow records.

The apartment was on the second floor of a grungy two-story typical Baltimore row house. There was a narrow flight of stairs to the landing and the door to the apartment had a lock that anyone could pick. Once inside, there was a little hallway off which there were four doorways: one to the kitchen, one to a bedroom, one to the bathroom and one to a living room. A second bedroom off the living room was mine. The kitchen overlooked a small backyard where some roses grew. A small wooden porch off the kitchen had stairs that led to the backyard.

Soon, we started a group cooking effort. Walter, Jack, Nancy and I and often Darrell Salk went to the Lexington market and looked around for all the best buys. We pooled our money to buy ingredients for the meals that we planned on the spot. The market was unlike almost any other in the US at the time. Stalls for everything fresh, pickled or smoked were under a huge roof. Unlike many farmers' markets, this market was open all year long. Once we got to know some of the butchers, we'd often get a break on a cut of meat. We came up with a schedule for each of us to be responsible for cooking a meal on one day and for doing the dishes on another day. We had a lot to learn.

One Saturday, I planned to make beef stew. Now I'm incredulous that I didn't consult a cookbook but back then I was confident to just guess. It couldn't be that hard. We had beef, potatoes, tomatoes, celery and carrots. Jack and I were alone that afternoon and everybody was coming over later. I figured that meat cooks quickly (like a steak on the grill) and potatoes, on the other hand, take a long time (like baked potatoes). I put a big pot on the stove, peeled and quartered the potatoes and put them in, to simmer. Then Jack and I went over to the Homewood campus to play squash. When we got back, the pot was full of a hot slurry of potato mush. Walter and Nancy came in and quickly figured out that dinner was going to be a disaster. I put in all the other ingredients and we waited until they were marginally done and

69

then we ate the tasteless, warm vichyssoise. The next time, I used a cookbook.

Jack didn't try to cook anything challenging for some time. Once we bought a ham steak that he was assigned to cook. We told him all he had to do was brown it on both sides in a frying pan. He took a chair and put it six inches from the stove, lit the burner, put the ham steak in the frying pan and sat down with his book – most likely something such as *Dune*. The rest of us went to the living room to watch the tube. Suddenly, we noticed this stream of smoke coming across the ceiling of the hallway and into the living room. I jumped up and ran to the kitchen to find Jack sitting quietly, completely absorbed in his book and the ham steak burning up next to him. From then on, he always cooked with a timer.

Jack had an incredible ability to focus every single bit of attention on the written word. While we played loud music with everybody talking to each other, Jack sat and read as if in another world. He remembered everything he read. I was surprised to find him reading *The Lord of the Rings* or *The Hobbit* for the hundredth time. For him, it was like playing a favorite Otis Redding album again even though he knew all the songs. He also *had* to read any written word that was in front of him. Sometimes at breakfast it was even hard to get his attention because his eyes had found the writing on a cereal box or juice carton.

We had similar views on the value of things. In a course on microbiology, we were required to inoculate mice with pneumococcus and then study their illness. Neither Jack nor I could understand why one would sacrifice these cute little mice for the sake of teaching medical students about pneumonia. We put them in our pockets and brought them back to 311 East 30th Street. Beula and Ruby. We put them in a bucket with some food and bedding and positioned the bucket next to our bed. We went to sleep in our single bed, which we were finding nicer and nicer. Suddenly, I was aware of a small creature crawling between the sheets. Whoa. The mice had gotten out. We put them back in the bucket, but we could hear them jumping – jumping again and again until bingo they reached the top and pulled themselves into the bed. We put a top on the bucket and the next day we went out and bought a big yellow plastic garbage can about 30 inches high. Beula and Ruby went into the can with their food and bedding. That night, I heard a persistent boink, boink, boink. As I looked and listened, I realized that Beula and Ruby were becoming Olympic jumpers. Instead of studying the effects of pneumococcus, we were studying how high mice could learn to jump if we gradually increased the height of their container! I couldn't fall asleep listening to them practice. Finally, Ruby reached the top of the 30-inch garbage can and came into the bed. I put her back into the can, but she was out almost immediately. The next day, we gave the garbage can a new role and put Beula and Ruby in a new home – a large fish tank with a top.

We hadn't actually assessed the sexual status of Beula and Ruby, but it became clear within a few weeks that Beula was a guy and that Ruby was expecting many baby mice. We had saved the mice and they had propagated. Now we had 12 mice – more than we could accommodate. We put up with them until the babies were full grown, but the tank was crowded and smelly and we feared that even more mice were on the way. Fortunately, it was spring, and we took them out to a local park and released all of them. A flurry of white dots scattered across the green lawn into the woods. I was ambivalent about the whole thing. On the one hand, we rescued the mice from pneumonia but, in the end, they were going to have to survive in the pretty brutal world of nature.

Most of the time, Jack and I saw eye to eye and got along easily, but of course we had times when we annoyed each other. Both of us could be stubborn. One weekend at the end of April, we all decided to go canoeing on the Potomac. The weather was hot for April, and we wanted to cool off on the water. We trooped down to a designated spot on the river where we could rent the canoes. Jack and I were in one canoe. The idea was to go downstream for several miles and then return up a canal that ran next to the river. Jack announced that he had learned how to canoe in summer camp and that he should be in the back. At first, I protested but he insisted that steering a canoe took finesse and experience and he had been trained to do this whereas I hadn't.

We started down the river. "Anne, switch sides?" he said. A little later I heard: "Anne, could you row faster and more consistently?" I was sweating like a pig. I turned my head to peer back at Jack who was calmly holding the paddle close to the back end of the canoe. Steering. I said, "why aren't you paddling?"

"Oh, I am. I was just adjusting our course for those rapids ahead."

Every time I looked around it was the same thing, Jack steering and me paddling. I started to get really pissed! I thought we were sharing something together. Now I'm the dog for his sled! I asked him why I was doing all the work and he said that he was working really hard too but somehow I was always looking back when he was steering. We got to the point where we had to turn around and go back up the canal. Now there was no steering involved, but Jack was still pulling the same trick. I jumped out of the canoe into the shallow water, smacked the paddle on the water and splashed him. Then I tipped him over into the water. He calmly turned the canoe upright and proceeded on. No matter how I screamed at him, he said he was sorry, but he clearly didn't think he had done anything wrong. We got back to the canoe rental place, and I went home without him and said, "I'm not talking to you again." That night he stayed at Walter's place.

Jack never apologized about the canoe. But he did say we shouldn't destroy a good thing over a stupid canoe ride. He said that we should just agree not to go out in a canoe again. After a week, I was able to forgive him. He moved back in again and we went back to our happy ways together. In hindsight, this was the worst argument we ever had. Essentially, I was having a temper tantrum and Jack just tried to ignore it as he did many times throughout our relationship.

After a year and three quarters, we had finished all our basic science courses, and I was ready for my clerkships. I was assigned to the Surgery Service for my first rotation. Needless to say, I anticipated seeing plenty of blood when cutting people open. I was terrified of this because I was frightened by blood and in high school I had fainted dead away at a medical demonstration at the University of Chicago. My first assignment was in the emergency room at Hopkins. It was always hopping, and, at the time, medical students could evaluate patients and sew up wounds with little supervision.

One afternoon a man was rushed into the emergency room, his yellow jumpsuit soaked in blood – the result of many stab wounds. He was taken right to the trauma bay. Another man who arrived at the same time had a forehead wound and I was assigned to sew him up. The wound was nearly a complete circle and the guy said that he had been struck with a coke bottle by the stabbed man in the trauma bay. Fortunately, the wound wasn't bloody. In fact, it was pink instead of red. Hmmm . . . strange. I got out the suturing kit and injected some lidocaine to numb the area. Before sewing though I probed the wound with my forceps. Uh oh! There was an irregular circular edge on the skull! What could it be? Could it be glass? Could the pinker blood mean that it was mixed with spinal fluid?

I called the surgeon over to take a look. "Better get a skull x-ray right away," he said as he looked over the wound.

The x-ray showed that two inches of a coke bottle had broken off and was sitting in his brain! I was feeling the end of the broken piece at the forehead. Despite the size of the wound, he was awake, coherent and outwardly normal. The lesson was: Don't depend on outward appearances or first impressions. As it turned out the stabbed man who was covered in blood had only superficial wounds but the guy who stabbed him needed brain surgery to remove the bottle from his right frontal lobe.

Another evening, I was sewing somebody up when a big hullabaloo arose and a woman with a dishtowel pressed to the side of her head was hustled behind a curtain around the gurney next to me. Several doctors went behind the curtain and shortly a man, who obviously knew her, rushed in with a glass mason jar. The man and woman had been making love and the man had bitten off the woman's ear in a fit of passion. He had brought the ear in the jar. Because the wound on the side of the woman's head had so many nasty bacteria as the result of a human bite, the doctors couldn't sew the ear back on until the wound healed. So, the surgeons peeled off the skin of the ear that had arrived in the jar and then tucked the cartilage in the woman's abdominal fat where it could survive for weeks. Later the ear was removed from the abdomen and successfully reattached. Such a cool technique to keep the cartilage of her ear alive waiting for the exterior wound to heal. Also, I was surprised to learn what people can do in their intimate moments.

I also had two weeks of experience in neurosurgery and for the first time I saw the living human brain. It was a beautiful, delicate, light white-pink substance with hills and canyons covered by a web of purple-blue veins and thin red arteries. It throbbed with the heartbeat. I was holding a retractor to hold back part of the brain when my vision suddenly turned yellowish, and I could only see in the center. I was fainting! I backed up quickly, gave my retractor to a nurse and sat down with my head between my knees. Phew! I had not lost consciousness. A career in surgery, however, was not in my future.

One morning in the middle of June 1971, Jack and I were having breakfast at the small round table in the kitchen. We'd been together for over a year now and I remember he was wearing his cutoffs and no shirt. Suddenly, he knelt down by my chair.

"Will you marry me?" he asked.

His sudden proposal was so cute. I loved him for it, but we had never talked about marriage before.

"I think it's a bad idea," I said. "I don't believe in marriage as a formal thing. What is the meaning of a piece of paper? Commitments are made by living them not by taking vows. We should just live together as we are doing."

Jack smiled but patiently explained, "I agree totally but I have these wonderful grandparents who will never understand. If we get married, we can just agree that it is a temporary thing between us. If we are married, then we can sleep together when we visit my family."

I didn't want to talk about whether it was temporary or not, but I did want to make sure he understood who his future wife wanted to be. "You have to realize, Jack, that I am a really driven woman and want to make real discoveries and go somewhere in the world. It will be hard on you because I am so aggressive and ambitious."

"Anne," he said. "I already know you are going to have a great career and I want to be part of it. Don't worry. I have enough sense of myself and my own worth that even if my wife is a driven woman, I can deal with that and be proud."

I called my parents and told them about our decision. They couldn't believe it. "You're only 23. Who is this Jack guy? What kind of family is he from?"

"Mom! He went to Dartmouth. He's a medical student. At Hopkins. How disreputable can that be?" I told them I was in love and we'd made up our minds. They knew they couldn't stop me.

"When are you actually going to get married?" asked my mother. Maybe she thought she could stall for time and if the date were far enough in the future, I'd change my mind.

"How about the end of July?"

"*The end of July?* That's only four weeks away."

"Okay, okay." I backed up. She had a point. "How about the beginning of August? August 7th? At our farm in Ohio. It won't take much. We'll just have family and a few friends."

"Anne. That's going to be harder than you think. You want it at the farm? Where will people stay?"

"Well, Jack's family can stay in Chillicothe and my friends will just bring tents and camp on the lawn." Chillicothe was the nearest real town 20 miles from the farm. The closest place with a motel or hotel.

"But there is only one bathroom in the farmhouse."

"So? It shouldn't be a problem." I was used to roommates and shared living spaces. Bathrooms were a minor technicality. "It's definitely the best time," I argued, "because I'm sure I can get the weekend off from my medicine rotation."

I heard a sigh. She couldn't argue with the busy schedule of a doctor-to-be. "What will we do about invitations? I'm not sure I can get them printed up in time."

"I'm going to draw a picture for the wedding invitation and we can just get it copied. Don't worry. I'll take care of it." I'd been tortured by my mother's demand that I attend formal teas, dinners, dancing school lessons, and the crowning achievement of a debutante ball – no way was I going to abide by such fussy traditions for *my* wedding.

"When can we meet him?" said my father. I hadn't brought him home earlier because I knew it would be an unpleasant experience for Jack and me. Besides, I really didn't care if they approved of him and I figured that they would likely try to dissuade me if they thought they could. I really liked Jack's family more than my own.

"We'll come to the farm in July."

We went to the farm and met my parents. They thought he was a bit quiet and too skinny. Jack couldn't believe how intense my parents were and how the dinner conversation always evolved into heated discussions of controversial topics.

"Don't your parents ever just make small talk?" Jack asked me later.

"I wish." I probably should have warned him in advance of my parents' habit of using the dinner table as a forum for their Socratic method to test his intellect. They baited Jack the entire visit and tried to find the limits of his knowledge about history and science. Temperamentally, Jack tried to avoid these confrontations, but the truth was that he knew more facts about not just medicine but astronomy, politics and history than they could handle. By the end of the visit, I could tell they were impressed with his quiet intelligence.

I made a pen-and-ink drawing of a piglet and hedgehog (quiet, shy, bearded and hairy) holding hands for the front of the invitation and sent them out (Figure 4.1). My mother worked

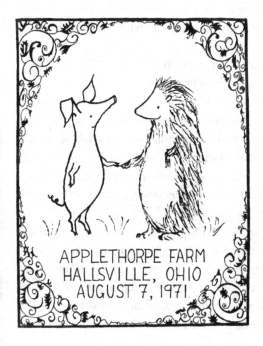

Figure 4.1 The wedding invitation.

APPLETHORPE FARM
HALLSVILLE, OHIO
AUGUST 7, 1971

harder than I realized behind the scenes to find a caterer who could arrange a dinner in Hallsville, Ohio. Not a mean feat. I wanted a two-layer cake with applesauce spice as one layer and chocolate as the other layer. I didn't want a traditional cake. The baker said that the cake would collapse. But he finally arranged to make it.

We found a pastor to perform the wedding, but we had to get counseling for it to be legal in Ohio. No way were we going to endure a session with a clergyman about the 'sacred commitment of marriage.' Besides, we didn't have time. Instead, we decided to get legally married in Maryland before the official wedding because in Maryland you could get a license with only one day's notice and no counseling. At lunch time, August 2, on our medicine rotations, we asked the senior residents if we could get a few hours off to go downtown and get married. They said "Really? You're just getting married at lunch time?"

We had bought simple gold wedding bands, and we were excited to complete this task so easily all while working hard on our rotations.

"Well, we guess you can have the afternoon off." They also gave us the Friday off before the wedding in Ohio.

Jack, Walter, Nancy Serrell and I drove out to Ohio on August 6, a Friday. Jack's family – his parents, brother, sister and her husband and little boy, Brian, and three grandparents arrived from New England. A few friends of Jack and mine from high school and college also came and set up tents on the lawn. My family, my parents, uncle and aunt, brother, sister and grandmothers were all there plus a few of my parents' friends and my godparents.

Ohio in August can be horribly hot and humid but by some miracle a front had come through on Thursday and the weather was absolutely perfect – cool, clear, blue and crisp. We all got up on Saturday and played croquet, went swimming in the pool, drank beer and hung out together on the lawn. At three o'clock, everybody went up to the farmhouse to get dressed. Jack wore tails and I wore

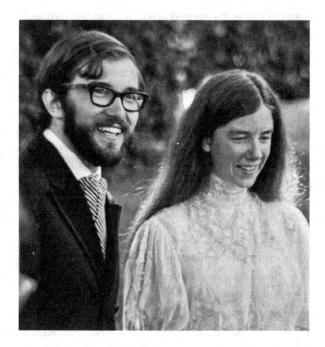

Figure 4.2 My wedding with Jack.

a white lace lawn dress (a shirt with a high collar and a long white skirt) that had belonged to my great grandmother. We all then went out on the lawn under the enormous sycamore tree and had a quick little wedding ceremony and it was done (Figure 4.2)! We had a great dinner and then cut the wedding cake that was decorated with two crossed scalpels. After dinner, Walter, Nancy, Jack and I drove to White Lake and got stoned and spent the night in a cabin before heading back to Baltimore.

Once we got back from the wedding, Jack moved into the old apartment with Nancy and me. We settled into the medical school rotations and bought our first pieces of furniture. The first was a couch of water buffalo leather from a Scandinavian store. The second was a full-size mattress. We had enough money to buy the mattress but not the frame. We went down to the lumber yard and bought some wood. When we got home, I fashioned a platform bed that we slept on for at least 10 years. Jack turned out to be no fix-it man. I had to teach him how to put new wires into a lamp, how to sink screws and drill holes. I had to teach him how to drive a stick shift car. I learned a lot about how things are put together by my father who could fix almost everything. On the other hand, Jack loved the same music, the same comic strips (*Doonesbury* and *Calvin and Hobbes*), sports and woods that I did. Both of us loved to walk silently through the woods and listen to the rustling leaves, the birds and shadows. Our relationship relied on being together. We were inseparable.

The rotation on the medicine service was nonstop work accompanied by constant humiliation. We had to learn about diseases of the heart, stomach, liver, kidneys, intestines and more. We were required to give every patient a complete workup, after which the senior professor demanded a list of the possible diseases that could account for the symptoms – what's called the differential diagnosis. In the beginning, I came up with only about three or four possibilities and was chided for such a short and incomplete list. Next time, my differential had 10 possibilities and I was told I had missed things and should work harder. No matter how hard I tried I never seemed to get any positive feedback. Punishment made me less likely to work hard whereas I lived for praise and encouragement. I concluded that medicine was *no* fun.

While I was rotating on medicine, however, I was assigned two neurology cases which were taught by the neurology professors. They found patients who were so absolutely fascinating. They showed how one could use a careful neurological examination to find out the location of the problem in the brain. The neurology professors were enthusiastic and supportive instead of punitive. One of the neurology residents, David Zee (who became one of the greats of neuro-ophthalmology), often found me on the medicine wards and took me to see some unusual patients. Neurology seemed to be a subspecialty of wonderful people who dealt with little blood, studied a beautiful brain and approached patient diagnoses as an opportunity to solve the puzzle of the patient's disease. Although neurology was then a subspecialty that took care of many untreatable diseases, I was completely captivated by the challenge to find more effective therapies.

In December, over Christmas break, Jack and I went on our 'honeymoon' to ski in Aspen, Colorado. Jack was a passionate skier. I liked to ski but I'd become afraid of heights and speed and moguls. Jack had learned to ski at a young age, and when he went to college he spent all his free time on the Dartmouth Skiway perfecting his short swing. He constantly bragged about the great skiing in the mountains of Vermont and New Hampshire. I'd grown up in Chicago so the most I did as a child was to make day trips to Wilmot Hills or Cascade Mountain – hardly more than ripples in the vast horizon of the plains. The next best thing was Iron Mountain in the Upper Peninsula or Boyne Mountain or Nubs Nob in upper lower Michigan. I had, however, made three trips to ski in the Rockies in high school. Two trips to Vail and one to Aspen. So, I teased Jack all the time about how Vermont and New Hampshire only had hills and that the real mountains were in the west. This was to be Jack's first trip to ski in the Rockies. He had been there in the summer as a child but never in the winter.

Aspen, at 8,000 feet, was nestled into a valley at the base of a large ski mountain with many lifts and ski runs. The town was older and had much more character than Vail or other popular ski resorts. Many buildings from the turn of the century still stood. Cultural events were year-round and the permanent population of about 5,000 ran small rustic hotels, restaurants and shops. We checked into a small hotel within walking distance of a lift.

The next morning, when we reached the top of the mountain, Jack was instantly in seventh heaven. He had never seen such fine snow and beautiful trails. Jack couldn't sing or dance but, on the slopes, he was incredibly graceful. With his short swing, he bobbed and weaved down the slopes in front of me to the next rise and then turned to watch me ski awkwardly and cautiously down to meet him. He was always very patient with me. He knew I was afraid to go too fast or out of control. I didn't want to break my neck the way my eighth-grade teacher had. Several times a day, however, he said that he was going to go down this or that black diamond trail and meet me at the bottom. He disappeared off the edge of a steep vertical slope and was gone from view. I took the easier blue run and found him waiting at the bottom. Going up the many ski lifts from time to time we passed small one-room cabins tucked among the trees. They were rustic, wood cabins with one or two small windows and a stovepipe on the outside. Once we skied down to examine one. It reminded me of Heidi's grandfather's cabin in the Alps I had read about as a child. I wished I could have a cabin like that when I got older. After that week of great skiing, Jack was convinced that skiing in the Rockies was something special and we vowed to do it again when we were able.

5

• • • • •

The Car Accident

I had finished all my required clerkships – just nine months – surgery, medicine, pediatrics, ob/gyn and psychiatry by the end of December 1971. Everything else was elective. Jack was training to be a real doctor by taking clinical rotations, including neurology, infectious disease, rheumatology, but I spoke with the dean of students who said that I could take a leave of absence from medical school and join the pharmacology department as a graduate student. When it was time to graduate with my medical school class, I could count the graduate work in pharmacology as elective courses and return from leave of absence just to graduate with the MD. The pharmacology department agreed to accept me as a graduate student and count my medical school coursework as fulfilling all the course requirements for the pharmacology PhD, with the exception of a few seminar courses that I had to take. I didn't know anybody else who designed their own combined degree program. All I had to do basically was complete my dissertation research satisfactorily and I would have both my MD and my

PhD. I got both agreements in writing. So, I officially became a pharmacology graduate student working in Sol Snyder's laboratory.

I was the first MD/PhD student to join Snyder's lab. The whole purpose of the combined degree program was to train clinical doctors in fundamental scientific investigation *and* clinical medicine so that they could eventually work at the interface between basic research and clinical patient care. A year after I started at Hopkins, the institution acquired an NIH grant to support an official combined degree program. Two male MD/PhD candidates began their graduate studies in Sol's lab. I remember asking one of them how to calculate the osmolality of a complex solution and he confidently gave me a formula to write down. Just to be sure, I asked the second guy the same question. He promptly gave me an entirely different formula. When I looked up the formula in my textbook, I realized they were both wrong. My little social science experiment made me realize that men were capable of confidently saying something without hesitation even if they were unsure of the answer. I also realized I was perfectly capable of finding out what I needed to know from more reliable resources.

Sol put me on a project to determine whether a substance called homocarnosine was a neurotransmitter. Homocarnosine is a dipeptide (two amino acids) made up of GABA and histidine. It is present in high concentration in the brain. What is it doing there? Where was it located in the cell? Was it released on stimulation? Was it split into GABA and histidine at the synapse? Was it inactivated by specific mechanisms? These were the questions I would have to answer if homocarnosine was to be considered a neurotransmitter.

To identify a new neurotransmitter or chemical messenger was quite an accomplishment so I wanted to pursue it, but I first had to develop an efficient way to measure it. All the existing measures for homocarnosine involved a lot of tissue and complex chromatography and electrophoresis. The process was very slow and inefficient. My first job was to invent what's called 'an assay,' which allowed me to measure the dipeptide accurately in up to 75 samples a day – a big number in those days. I was just starting to look at different potential methods and things were going well when Jack and I, Walter and another couple made plans to go winter camping on the Appalachian Trail one weekend.

We called the park service and reserved a lean-to about two miles from the road at the point where the trail crossed at Harpers Ferry. I had a new parka and we all had good sleeping bags, boots, gaiters, cooking gear and food. The night before it had snowed but that seemed to make our adventure even more fun, and we headed out in Piglet in the morning. The snow was about 20 inches deep, but we knew the walk was relatively short and decided to go for it. The first portion was steep, and the going was difficult but one of us broke trail and the rear positions were relatively easy. When we reached the lean-to, we discovered it had collapsed under the weight of the snow and lay in ruins. There was no shelter if we stayed the night so after a bit of debate we decided to hike back and return to Baltimore.

We arrived back at 311 East 30th Street around 6 p.m. and decided to order pizza from Pecora's on Greenmount Ave. We turned on the TV and Ben Hur was playing; everyone was happy. I had seen Ben Hur on my eleventh birthday and fainted from the bloody chariot scene so figured I'd be better off picking up the pizza. I hopped into Piglet and tootled down the few blocks to Greenmount Ave, turned left and swung into a parking place just opposite Pecora's restaurant. That's when I saw a cop car parked right in front of the pizza place with a cop inside who was looking right at my license plates. Damn! The plates had expired, and I was afraid he was going to nail me. To avoid him, I averted my eyes, figuring that if I made no eye contact, he would have to leave his cozy cruiser to find me in the store. I opened the car door, got out and looked down at the pavement as I closed the door and stepped out into the street.

Wham! Before I knew what was happening, I felt my left leg stunned and I was flipping up over a car, sliding down off the trunk and onto the street. The cop was out of the car in an instant and came over to where I was lying on the pavement, my hand finding the abnormal bend in my thigh. A crowd was staring down at me, including the poor young man and his girlfriend whose car had hit me. She was crying and sobbing. I told the policeman to call my husband at 353–8266. I tried to raise my head but couldn't because my blood was frozen to the street. The ambulance arrived and I was loaded onto a gurney. My leg was obviously fractured and now it was beginning to hurt. I asked the EMTs to take me to Johns Hopkins, but they refused saying that they were required to take me to the closest emergency room – Union Memorial, known as the hospital from hell.

I arrived in the ER, bleeding, with a broken leg. My new parka was all stained with dirt and blood. The doctor cut off my favorite seasoned pair of blue jeans and began to check me out. I kept asking everyone who came near me to call Jack. I was given a shot of Demerol and the pain eased. They could only find the large gash at the back of my head and the broken left femur.

Finally, they called Jack. He and everyone else had wondered where the hell Anne and the pizza were. They were starving. They stopped at Pecora's and picked it up on the way to the hospital.

The doctor in the ER was a moonlighting Hopkins resident. He said they had to admit me because the femur fracture required traction and either surgery or a full-body cast. Besides, they had to watch me for internal injuries. The next day, Dr. Mulholland, an orthopedic surgeon, came to see me; Jack had called someone at Hopkins who said Mulholland was supposed to be okay. Mulholland suggested that he could put what's called a Kuntscher nail down the middle of my thigh bone since it was a simple fracture with only one loose fragment. The nail held the pieces together while they healed. This procedure would get me back on crutches in three weeks and walking with a cane in six to eight weeks. The alternatives were miserable: six months in traction or six months in a body cast from below my knee to above my hip. Forget that! I might be woozy from the Demerol, but I had research to do and a PhD to get. I chose the nail – an 18-inch piece of titanium that would be inserted at the top of the femur and driven down the inside to the knee.

Surgery was scheduled for the next day. Jack and two friends visited me in the evening. I got a shot of Demerol every four hours. I was drifting in and out. I remarked how odd it was that little things were flying across my field of view. No one thought much of it. That night, my roommate called the nurse twice to tell her that my breathing sounded funny. The nurse checked me and told my roommate not to worry.

When Jack came in to see me before I went to surgery, he found me in four-point restraints – each limb in a leather strap tied to the bedpost. A group of nurses and doctors surrounded my bed. I had pulled out my IV and my bladder catheter. I had bitten one of the nurses. I was incoherent and gasping for breath. The doctors asked Jack how much I drank. Maybe I had an alcohol disorder and was in DTs (delirium tremens). I was agitated, with a racing pulse and rapid breathing. Finally, someone drew a blood gas directly from a large artery – a measurement of how much oxygen I had. My oxygen level was very low, and my chest x-ray showed a white-out – a sign of fluid, infection or blood in the lungs. Petechiae – tiny hemorrhages of blood under the skin – were noted under my eyelids and in my fingernail beds.

Surgery was canceled, and I was taken to the Intensive Care Unit. I had fat emboli. When long bones such as the femur are broken, toxins from the marrow leak into the bloodstream and cause fats in the blood to form little globs or clots that then fly out to the ends of blood vessels clogging them up and causing small hemorrhages all over the body and brain. My lungs couldn't absorb oxygen. My brain was damaged by the emboli and was even worse because of the low oxygen. They gave me huge doses of steroids in the hope of saving me. At Jack's request, Richard Johnson, the senior neurologist we knew at Johns Hopkins, came over and examined me. He took Jack aside and told him that things were pretty grave and that only 25–50 percent of people survived this. My parents came to visit. The situation was dire.

After about two days, things began to improve. My first recollection was of seeing a group of doctors faraway down a long corridor, chatting pleasantly together. Jack was at my side, his hand resting on my arm. I knew he was out to kill me! For that matter everyone else was also! He told me he loved me and that things were going to be okay. What a bunch of bullshit. He was poisoning me. As I improved, I could recognize rationally that everybody was trying to help me and loved me, but the emotional side of my brain stepped in and pointed out that all this nice stuff was just a façade trying to cover up all the evil underneath. Jack later told me that I had been belligerent, pulling at all my restraints, and even after I calmed down, I was never the same. It took weeks for the overt paranoia to wear off but there was a permanent paranoid undercurrent that is still with me. Just as I had had emboli to my lungs, I had also had emboli to my brain which must have caused damage.

Back on the floor several days later, the nurses watched over me more carefully, but they were still seemingly afraid and unhelpful. My leg was in traction, and they had to wait a couple of weeks while my lungs and brain improved before they could put the nail in my leg. I was very anemic as I had lost several units of blood into my thigh, and I had several transfusions. One night, the bandages holding my leg in the splint became unraveled and I called the nurse to come help me rebandage it. The broken leg was hanging uncomfortably at an angle. The nurse said that they had strict orders not to manipulate the leg as more fat emboli might 'fall' out. How ridiculous. I asked her to call the house officer who confirmed his unwillingness to help. I called Jack, who came right over and helped me get my leg back safely and comfortably in the supporting bandages. Two weeks later, the leg was finally pinned with a Kuntscher nail, and I was soon discharged on crutches.

Within five weeks of the accident, I was back in the lab. I used a cane to get around, but the real trouble was whenever I entered the corridor from the lab, I was sure that a speeding car, person or unidentifiable object would run me down.

The homocarnosine project that I'd first started at Sol's suggestion was working out, but my enthusiasm for it was lagging because my data suggested it was unlikely to be a neurotransmitter. I could pursue it, but it wasn't exciting, and I felt like it was a failure. I spent time, though, collecting enough data to be able to publish a paper on my new method of measuring homocarnosine. Previous techniques for measuring homocarnosine were time-consuming and required the use of large amounts of tissue. My procedure was specific and sensitive enough to detect as little as 0.1 nmol of tissue homocarnosine. I could measure up to 75 tissue samples in a single day. Nevertheless, pursuing a dead end was just not worth it. Now that we knew that homocarnosine was unlikely to be a neurotransmitter, it was better to start a new investigation. I decided to look at potential side projects just to see what might be interesting enough to pursue. Throughout my time in the lab so far, I had attended the weekly neurology grand rounds and neuropathology conferences. Seeing the patients' sufferings in the hospital and hearing about neuropathology work done by other scientists continued to make me want to discover more transmitters for the key pathways. Intellectually, it was exciting.

Emotionally, it would be so rewarding if we could offer patients more treatment help. I thought of my pioneer ancestors cutting down trees to make rafts to float from Ohio to New Orleans and building the first grain elevators in Chicago when it still looked like a swamp. Maybe I had inherited some of their fortitude and imagination. Certainly I shared their enthusiasm for exploring the unknown.

Around that time, I first met Candace Pert. A year and a half earlier, when she was a new graduate student in pharmacology, she had taken over and finished the project about histamine I had worked on during my summer rotation. We had published an article about it in *Science*. I was the first author. Now our lab benches were right across from each other, so we had a lot of chances to interact. Candace was fun to talk to, always enthusiastic about her work and very smart. Although we were the only two women students in the lab, we were opposites in appearance. I dressed in jeans and gym shoes whereas she dressed in low-cut short cotton shifts. She had had a son when she was a college student whom she often brought to the lab, where she kept him busy putting caps on the scintillation vials. Her husband, Agu Pert, was a behavioral neuroscientist who worked on the effects of nerve gas on monkeys at Edgewood Arsenal, which at the time was the home of the country's chemical and biological weapons program.

Lab rotations were required of pharmacology graduate students and Candace picked a two-month rotation in a lab down the hall from Sol's lab run by Professor Pedro Cuatrecasas, another faculty pharmacologist. He had worked out methods for measuring insulin and other hormone receptors, and Candace brought back the strategy to measure receptors to Sol's lab.

Pedro found that insulin could be labeled with [^{125}I] (a radioactive isotope of iodine) to a very high specific activity – essentially meaning that nearly every molecule of insulin had the [^{125}I] label. Pedro incubated membranes from various body organs with the labeled radioactive insulin and then filtered the samples and rinsed off any unbound insulin. The amount of [^{125}I]-insulin bound to the membranes reflected the number of insulin receptors in a particular tissue. This was a fine way to label a protein like insulin, but much smaller molecules or drugs couldn't be labeled with [^{125}I] without altering the action of the drug.

So instead, Candace first obtained a sample of morphine labeled with [^{3}H] tritium. Tritium is a weak radioactive form of hydrogen. Candace used Pedro's new strategies to isolate the receptor in the brain for morphine. Her first experiments using [^{3}H]-morphine didn't work. Not enough of the drug bound to brain membranes. Next, she tried the opiate antagonist [^{3}H]-naloxone, which *did* bind tightly to brain membranes and could be displaced by high concentrations of morphine. Naloxone was known even then to reverse the effects of opiate overdose. I remember the afternoon she first found the method to work! She turned to me and said, "Anne, I think I just discovered the way to measure opiate receptors in the brain! Let's go get a beer!" Sure enough, her method continued to work.

Just three months after my car accident, I went into the shower to wash my hair and as I was combing it huge handfuls fell into my hands. By the time I was ready to go to the lab, I had collected a brown sandwich bag full of hair. Jack and I were mystified. Surely this was a sign that something was wrong. I went to the student health center at the hospital. The nurse inquired loudly as to what the problem was, and I said I wanted a referral to a dermatologist because my hair was falling out. Chuckles emanated from the various people in the waiting room. I looked like I had a perfectly good head of hair. The nurse informed me I needed a referral from a doctor to see a specialist.

"I see you're worried that your hair is falling out," said the middle-aged doctor from the other side of a large desk. "You know, my dear," he began, sounding like an all-knowing father speaking to an ignorant teen overly concerned about her appearance, "everybody's hair falls out to a certain degree. It's natural. Don't worry."

"I know *some* hair falls out! But this much?" I opened the bag. "This much fell out this morning!" I could see him suppress a flinch as he struggled to keep his cool.

"Yes, yes. Even that much." I took the bands off my pigtails.

"You mean this much?" I ran my fingers through my hair and then held up the hundreds of strands of hair that covered my fingers to show him what I meant. Why wouldn't he listen to me? He was resolute against a silly hysterical woman medical student trying to overrule his authority and refused to make a referral.

What a jerk. I will never forget his arrogance, ignorance and chauvinism. I limped up to the dermatology floor with my cane and stopped one of the faculty in the hallway. I asked him if he knew what might be happening to my hair. He noticed my cane and asked about it. I told him about the accident and the fat emboli and the steroids. He asked when the accident occurred, and I told him it had been three months.

"Perfect," he said. "It's a telogen effluvium. It is not that uncommon. All the hair on your body has a life cycle and some are in the growing phase, anagens, and some are ready to fall out, telogens. Usually about 90 percent of your hair is in the anagen phase and about 10 percent in the telogen phase. When some people have a high fever, pregnancy, trauma or steroids, the anagens all go into shock and become telogens. It takes about three months for new hairs underneath to push out the telogens and that's what is happening today. It's hard to say how much hair you will lose but it should grow back."

What a relief! He predicted it to a T. If the first doctor had observed me carefully, asked questions and, most of all, taken me seriously, would he have diagnosed the problem properly? If I had not been a medical student, would I have had the confidence or vocabulary to stop another doctor in the hall and talk to him directly? Within several weeks, about half my hair had fallen out. It was diffuse, not patchy, so it didn't look grotesque. Then a new set of shorter fuzz started in and gradually filled in the missing hair. It was quite the 'do' – 2-inch hair and 18-inch hair.

That June, Jack, Nancy and I drove back out to Harpers Ferry and walked up the first steep slope of the trail. Jack carried most of the stuff since I was still walking with a cane. There was a beautiful ledge about 20 feet wide at the top of the slope where we pitched our tent high above the confluence of the Potomac and Shenandoah rivers. It was a lot more fun and beautiful than sleeping in the lean-to in the snow.

6

• • • • •

Neurotransmitters, Drugs and Receptors

Our apartment got to feeling small and Jack and I wanted a real room. We loved Nancy, however, and wanted to continue living with her. We looked around and found a place on 1631 Ingram Ave outside the city, in a middle-class neighborhood that lacked the raunchy character of our old apartment. It was a split townhouse and we were renting half – a basement that served as our kitchen/dining/laundry room, a first-floor living room that had a bedroom/bath and an upstairs with another bedroom and bath. Nancy took the upstairs bedroom; Jack and I had the first-floor bedroom. That gave everyone enough privacy and togetherness. We painted and wallpapered a large amount of the place and then enjoyed it. Nancy brought home the recipe for Chinese curried pork chops from her sister-in-law and they became a favorite of ours. Jack made many pumpkin pies for Halloween. He was also the breakfast guy, becoming an expert in pancakes and buckwheat sourdough waffles. We were a happy household.

After spending many afternoons in the library reading about previous studies on amino acids, I thought maybe I could find a way to measure receptors for GABA and glycine. GABA is a unique amino acid not found in proteins but present in high concentration in the brain. Glycine, on the other hand, is the simplest amino acid and is present in all proteins. How could this simple amino acid be a neurotransmitter? Based on my reading and digging up reports of old experiments, I realized there was evidence that the deadly plant neurotoxin known as strychnine blocked a part of the knee reflex. The knee reflex is when the doctor taps the tendon below your kneecap with her reflex hammer and your leg shoots out (from stimulation of the motor nerve to the thigh muscle) and then relaxes. When strychnine is given, the leg shoots out but isn't able to relax. In larger doses, the person goes into generalized muscle spasms and convulsions and stops breathing. A different group of scientists, not studying strychnine, had suggested that glycine was a neurotransmitter involved in triggering the relaxation phase of the knee reflex. When squirted onto the surface of a spinal motor neuron, glycine decreased the activity of the neuron. Glycine concentrations were high in parts of the spinal cord regulating reflexes.

I hypothesized that strychnine worked the way it did because it was binding to the glycine neurotransmitter receptor. It prevented glycine activating its receptor to block the firing of nerves to the thigh muscles and allowing the knees to relax. If I was right, I would have discovered something new about the lock (receptor) for the key (glycine). Demonstrating a specific glycine receptor would also provide important evidence that glycine, the simplest amino acid, was a neurotransmitter. Finding the glycine receptor would also have implications for our understanding of spasticity suffered by people with spinal cord disease and injury. I talked to Sol about my speculations, and he encouraged me to pursue it. However, to test my hypothesis, and measure whether strychnine is bound to glycine receptors, I had to get a sample of radioactive strychnine and purify it. That would be some work.

I sent off a 50 mg sample of powdered strychnine to be labeled with tritium by New England Nuclear Corporation and received back a small glass vial labeled 5 mCi (millicuries – a unit of radioactivity equal to one-thousandth of a curie – 3.7×10^7 disintegrations per second) of [^{3}H]-strychnine. They had replaced the regular hydrogen in the strychnine with radioactive tritium. The problem was that the vial was full of a disgusting, cloudy, greenish mix, most of which was unwanted. I had to purify the radioactive strychnine by separating it away from the gunk. Purifying it in the lab, however, required doing sequential chromatography, each run lasting six to eight hours. I didn't want to actually stay in the lab overnight. I liked to sleep at home with Jack.

So why not take it home? Back then we were much more casual about safety. We even pipetted radioactive liquids by mouth using a rubber tube attached to one end of the pipette and the other to a plastic mouthpiece. I wasn't too worried about taking a large amount of radioactivity home. It was dark when I pulled Piglet into the space behind our apartment, unloaded four dark brown glass gallon jugs of toxic chemicals (n-butanol, glacial acetic acid, methanol and chloroform), some glass equipment and the ugly vial of green liquid containing 5 millicuries of radioactive strychnine. I took it all into the downstairs kitchen, where I set up the equipment on the table. I applied a line of some of the radioactive, green stuff an inch from the bottom of a thin gel on a plastic sheet. I put the plastic sheet between two glass plates. I then set up a glass tray with a mix of the flammable and toxic liquids from the gallon jugs and immersed the bottom end of the plastic sheet in the liquid in the tray (Figure 6.1). It took five hours for the liquid to diffuse up the sheet and separate the greenish cloudy mix from the radioactive strychnine. Fumes were all over the apartment. When I was done, the strychnine purified, I dumped all the liquid solvents and residual radioactivity down our drain as we did in the lab. In today's world, we would never do such a thing but back then, although it would not

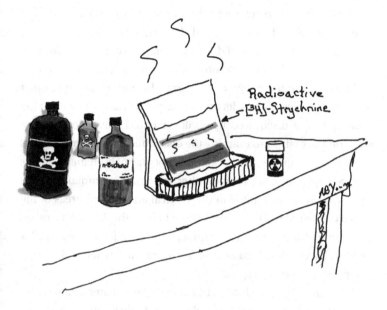

Figure 6.1 The thin layer chromatography setup I brought into our kitchen in Baltimore.

I applied a line of radioactive material at the bottom of a very thin gel on a plastic sheet. The sheet was put between two glass plates and then immersed in liquid solvents in the glass tray. After hours, the line of diffusion had risen almost to the top and the radioactive strychnine formed a separate line. Fumes were smelled throughout the house.

have been officially approved, I just figured I could speed up my research without getting caught.

Eventually, my experiments demonstrated that [³H]-strychnine would, in fact, bind to rat spinal cord membranes and could be blocked by glycine. I ground up the rat tissue and purified the membranes. I then added [³H]-strychnine either with or without excess glycine. These samples were then centrifuged, the resulting membrane pellets dissolved and the radioactivity in the pellet measured in a scintillation counter. Using my method, I examined all the properties of the glycine receptor. What solutions were best for measuring the receptors? What amount of tissue was needed in each sample? How quickly did the $[^3H]$-strychnine bind to the receptor and how quickly did it come off? If glycine could displace bound $[^3H]$-strychnine, what other amino acids could also do so?

I was exhilarated by the experiments. I could do an experiment every day and get the results the next day. The harder I worked, the more quickly I discovered new information. I was able, within a short period of time, to examine the distribution and characteristics of the receptor in the nervous systems not only of humans, primates and rats but also of snakes and other species. In mammals, glycine receptors are concentrated in the cervical and lumbar areas of the spinal cord where all the reflexes come in from the limbs. Snakes, on the other hand, have no arms and legs and therefore have no reflex like the knee reflex. Snakes have a consistent low level of glycine receptors all along the spinal cord.

These discoveries helped to understand how an important spinal cord reflex works. I began to wonder if and how the glycine receptor might be affected in spinal diseases such as spasticity.

Candace submitted her first paper on the opiate receptor to *Science* in December 1972 and it was published in March 1973. When her results were made public, TV and newspaper reporters swarmed the lab. Sol and Candace had many press interviews.

I was seven months behind Candace in my work, submitting my first paper in June 1973 to the *Proceedings of the National Academy of Sciences*. Submission required a sponsor who was a member of the National Academy of Sciences. Sol wasn't friends with any NAS members at that time. I asked my father if his friend Cheves Walling, a professor of chemistry at Columbia University, was a member and if he might help me. Cheves, who I also knew, agreed to sponsor my paper. It was published in October. However, no newspaper or TV reporters showed up at the lab for interviews.

The big difference, of course, was that people *cared* about the opiate receptor, but nobody had ever heard of glycine and GABA receptors. Opiate receptors have to do with pain relief, pleasure, reward and addiction – compelling and problematic issues that affect most people in their everyday lives. Glycine and GABA are about reflex control and inhibition in the nervous system, which are not key issues for the average, healthy person. Candace had found the receptor for opium, one of the oldest drugs used by humans. Just a year or so later, it was discovered that the body could make its own opiates: endorphins and enkephalins. At meetings, when we walked around together, she was surrounded by admirers. Her no-bra, short dresses look was as sexy as her opiate research. I was just a sidekick. My jeans and work shirt look was as plain as my discoveries about the spinal cord. I might have felt envious of the attention she received, but there was no question that Candace's work was groundbreaking, and I had seen firsthand how she had put her heart and soul into her experiments.

Writing papers with Sol was amazingly productive. When I met with him to discuss my data, he often said, "Let's write it up." Then he pulled out a Dictaphone recorder from his desk, turned it on and said, "Okay, how should we start?" Talking back and forth, we dictated a draft: Introduction, Results and Discussion. I wrote up the Materials and Methods and prepared the figures and a list of references. Sol's secretary typed it all up. A paper could be completed in less than two weeks. Of course in those days, there was no internet or online data. I had to go to the library to hunt down references. Being dyslexic, this work went slowly and kept me in the library for many hours tracking down obscure publications on the knee reflexes and spinal pathways.

The lab could be a competitive place. The results of the experiments in my and Candace's studies depended on measuring levels of radioactivity in multiple samples. The number of experiments one could do depended on the number of measurements one could make. The main goal was to fill up the scintillation counters with vials of radioactive samples from our receptor experiments in order to keep the machines running 24 hours a day. Sol gave Candace a technician to help with her experiments. The technician came in at 5:30 a.m., did experiments and filled up the scintillation counters with vials before 8:30 a.m. In order to get my samples counted each day, I also began to come in at 5:30 a.m. to compete with Candace's technician to fill at least one scintillation counter. Eventually, we agreed to try to maximize results for both of us.

My experiments were going well, and in no time I had lots of data showing that you could label glycine receptors with tritiated strychnine. Supported by a fellowship from the Scottish Rite Foundation and then by a federal grant for training MD/PhD students, I began studying the pharmacology and structural qualities of the receptors. Although the opiate work got most of the attention, Sol featured my work at meetings as well and he gave me a technician to help my work go faster. I soon had 13 publications, including the first measurements that anyone had taken of the GABA receptor.

One night, Jack came home from working in neurovirologist Robert Herndon's laboratory. He told me about a graduate student who was studying a virus that could selectively kill a particular type of nerve cell (the granule cell) in the part of the brain called the cerebellum (which controls movement and balance). No other nerve cells in the structure were damaged by the virus.

"Wow!" I said to myself as well as to Jack. My curiosity was piqued. A question immediately popped into my mind. "Maybe I can discover the neurotransmitter of the granule cells."

With the exception of dopamine cells, I didn't know of any other situation in which a specific type of nerve cell in a structure could be killed while all the other cells around it remained intact. At the time, methods for killing one selective group of nerve cells didn't exist. So it was curious that a virus could do that. The cerebellar granule cells formed a prominent layer of cells that physiologists had found to be excitatory. I sensed a unique opportunity.

What was the best and easiest way to proceed? One approach would be to measure potential neurotransmitter levels in the animals with missing granule cells compared to controls. This would be a complex series of experiments using many animals. One feature common to all the potential neurotransmitters was a pump system that could act at very tiny concentrations such as those in the synaptic cleft after neurotransmitter release. The pumps could be measured for all the accepted neurotransmitters such as norepinephrine, serotonin, dopamine and GABA. Pumps also exist for all amino acids because they are necessary for cells to function and make proteins. Could the pumps also *inactivate* the amino acid neurotransmitters once released from the nerve? The lab had found that if you made a preparation of tiny pinched-off synaptic nerve endings, called synaptosomes, and measured the pumps for amino acids, glutamate, aspartate and glycine had a high affinity pump that worked very quickly at very tiny concentrations such as the type of concentrations that were in the synapse after the endings' activation. Perhaps the three amino acids with the second high affinity pumps were neurotransmitters?

Officially, I was working on the glycine receptor in Sol's lab, but I thought that applying my methods to see if I could determine the specific neurotransmitter of this group of nerve cells would be a great, self-contained side project.

I talked to the anatomy graduate student in the lab where Jack was working. Mary Lou Oster-Granite and I already knew each other because we had been in the same anatomy foursome dissecting a human cadaver three years before. She was excited by my hypothesis and we designed three experiments that could be conducted over three weekends to try to identify the transmitter of the cerebellar granule cell.

The first weekend, Mary Lou gave me two hamster litters – one litter of normal animals and another whose cerebellar granule cells were deficient (nearly completely missing). I made a preparation of synaptosomes from the cerebella of each litter and measured the high affinity uptake of 12 amino acids, choline, serotonin, norepinephrine and GABA. We found that glutamate and aspartate were the only compounds affected – everything else was normal. The results were surprisingly clear, but more evidence was necessary. If the granule cells themselves were lost, I expected that the *number* and not the *potency* of the pump would be altered.

The next weekend, we measured the number and affinity (potency) of the amino acid uptake systems. We found that the number but not the affinity of glutamate and aspartate uptake was very reduced. This loss of the number of uptake sites was consistent with the loss of the number of granule cells. So now the final question was: Is the transmitter glutamate or aspartate? To find out, I had to measure the actual levels of the amino acids in normal cerebella and compare them to cerebella missing granule cells.

The third weekend I ground up the cerebella of one normal litter and the cerebella from a litter of animals with missing granule cells and ran both samples over an old-time amino acid analyzer that took all night for just one sample. Only glutamate levels were changed, not aspartate, thus consistent with the conclusion that glutamate is the likely neurotransmitter of cerebellar granule cells.

This set of experiments was the first to provide biochemical evidence that glutamate was the neurotransmitter of a particular nerve cell in the mammalian brain. We published the paper with me, Mary Lou, Robert Herndon (Mary Lou's supervisor) and Sol as coauthors. To this day I am proud of its design as a cool, clear study with significant findings. We had solved part of the puzzle of how the cerebellum works.

By now, Jack had started his internship at Baltimore City Hospital, and we had to move from the townhouse we shared with Nancy into resident apartments on the hospital grounds because he had to be on-site and call was every third night. Jack ate every chance he got because he was always worried he'd miss a meal. He gained 10 pounds to an all-time high of 160 pounds. We had my sister's cat Dickens who was just like a dog and greeted us at the door when we got home and woke us up in the morning by sitting on my face. The place had a big living room and one bedroom. The kitchen had giant cockroaches that sounded like scurrying mice in the cabinets and ate our cereal right out of the box.

I had plenty of material to write my thesis and my committee was pleased with my progress, so I started writing it up. Once I knew things were going well, we started planning for my internship and Jack's residency. Sol had done his internship in San Francisco and raved about what a great city it was. University of California San Francisco (UCSF) also had an outstanding neurology program. During his vacation, Jack and I went for a visit.

Neither of us had ever been to California. As soon as we got off the plane, we were blown away. It was gorgeous, the weather was great and the fog was mesmerizing. We interviewed for my internship and Jack's residency, and then we went camping up in Yosemite, hiking up to Little Yosemite Valley, where we camped for several days. We drove up the coast, which was shockingly beautiful. We stopped in Portland to visit Les on the commune where she was living.

"Totally hip," she boasted about her new lifestyle on a rabbit farm. "You use all the parts of the rabbit. Nothing is wasted. The meat is eaten. The fur is used for clothes. And the shit is used to grow earthworms that can then be sold for bait."

She showed us around the commune. All the rabbits lived in a big barn. The commune raised the rabbits and the earthworms and then sold the rabbits to processors and the worms to bait shops. Jack and I were really amazed at what a freaky scene it was – the huge, long barn filled with rabbits in cages over the expanse of rabbit droppings. Les had a girlfriend, and we all went out to a lesbian bar that night where Jack was the only guy. He took it all in stride. We slept in the hay loft of a barn on the farm and left the next day to go to the Olympic Peninsula.

Although Jack applied for neurology residency programs at Hopkins, Massachusetts General Hospital and UCSF, we both wanted more than anything to match to UCSF. On match day, Jack got calls accepting him into all the programs and so he signed up for UCSF. I applied to all the possible San Francisco hospitals for an internship. UCSF's medical program was the best and was very competitive. Since I hadn't done anything but the basic rotations and hadn't been on the wards for more than two years, I was hardly a prime candidate. I hadn't even done a neurology rotation. I didn't get into UCSF for an internship, but I did get an internship at Mount Zion Hospital, a decent community hospital with an acceptable medical teaching service.

I now had to finish up if I was going to be done in time for the internship and do one month of clinical work with Jack at Baltimore City Hospital in order to refresh my memory about how to give patients physical exams and other things too. I wrote my thesis on all my glycine receptor work. This was before the days of PCs or word processors, so I had to have someone type the manuscript. There couldn't be any mistakes. As I wrote, I xeroxed the text from time to time. One evening as I was leaving the lab at about nine at night, I carried my thesis, along with a book of Sol's on receptors, in a nice leather briefcase. I was wearing my usual jean jacket, where I kept my money and IDs in a pocket. I always walked to my car that was parked several blocks away in the slum that surrounded Johns Hopkins Hospital. Suddenly, a kid flashed out of an alley and grabbed my briefcase. I tried to hold on but he ripped it away even though I shouted, "All my money's in my pocket. You can have it. Just give me back the briefcase." He disappeared over a wall, taking two-thirds of my thesis; I only had a copy of the first third. I was going to have to do a lot of rewriting.

For weeks, I fumed. I thought about designing an aerosol bomb that could be linked to a briefcase lock. It contained garlic oil and methylene blue. Any kid stealing a briefcase would definitely be deterred afterwards, since turning purple from the methylene blue and stinking to high heaven from the garlic oil was pretty awful.

Candace and I both defended our theses on the same day, and we were both successful. The head of the pharmacology department and several senior faculty, however, called me into the office:

"We would like you to spend another year in the program before getting your PhD. If you get the degree a year after your MD, it will look like Hopkins doesn't have a rigorous program."

I couldn't believe it. They wanted to hold me back because they worried about what it would look like? "I already have 13 publications on my work and that's nothing to sneer at."

"We recognize what a fine job you have done but we also have to consider the future reputation of the program."

"I have already signed a contract to begin my internship on July 1 – a month from now."

"We will call the program director and try to have it deferred."

I was furious. "If you recall, both the dean and you agreed in writing to my plan for my MD/PhD program. I still have the letters from both of you. You know I don't need your PhD! I've already developed a reputation based on my work and I will just count the year as a fellowship! I'll drop off the government funded program and I'll spread the word to any applicants to the program that you are a bunch of liars."

I stood up, walked out of the office and slammed the door! Oh shit! What have I done? I went quickly down to Sol's office and told him the news.

The next day, the head of the department came to tell me that they had changed their mind and that I could graduate. But they made sure they wouldn't let anyone else graduate on such a fast track.

7

• • • • •

Training in Disorderly Movements

Jack and I moved to San Francisco. We subleased an apartment on Pine Street near Mt. Zion from a resident who was spending three months out of town. Jack loved neurology. He found it so much more interesting than general medicine. When he came home, he couldn't wait to tell me about all the cool patient cases he'd seen. He loved San Francisco General Hospital the best because exciting cases came in by ambulance right off the street. You had to be on your toes because it was frequently a matter of life and death for the patients.

I struggled through the first two months of my internship because I didn't know any medicine and the whole doctor thing was a mystery to me anyway. But I didn't really have a choice; a one-year internship in general medicine was required before starting neurology residency. Nevertheless, I eventually got the hang of it. It wasn't like lab science where success depended on imagination and hard work carrying out experiments. Medicine was formulaic. You had to try not to kill anyone, and mistakes were easy to make in the middle of the night. Overnight call was freaky, too. If things were slow enough, I could catch a little sleep in the call room, appropriately named because I had to answer whatever calls came in. When I got calls from the nurses, I could never figure out whether I was awake or dreaming. Once, I got to the call room about 4 a.m., stripped and got into bed. I woke up about an hour later and saw a five-foot spider spanning the walls and ceiling in the corner. My heart was racing! I jumped up and ran out into the hall stark naked! I couldn't stay in the hall, and I couldn't go back in the room with that spider. After about 10 minutes, I settled down and went back into the room realizing that the spider was just a bad dream. Thank God nobody had come into the hall.

I applied to UCSF and Stanford for neurology residency. As I mentioned, I hadn't even done a neurology rotation in medical school, so UCSF said they didn't think they could take me. I convinced Sol, Dick Johnson and others, however, from Hopkins to vouch for me and to tell UCSF how very interested I was in neurology and neuroscience despite never having done a neurology rotation and that I had already made important scientific contributions. Finally, UCSF accepted me into their program. Thank God.

Jack and I bought a house up at the top of 10th & Pacheco with down payment money I had been given over the years by my grandmother. The woman who owned the house had decorated it in raspberry and green. The kitchen was green with yellow tile. It smelled of her and her little white dogs. We worked on the house on our days off and in the evenings. We redid the whole inside except the dining room that had wallpaper we liked. Our biggest project was making a mantelpiece for the fireplace. We decided to use black walnut. I consulted my father on design, and Jack and I put together a simple but beautiful piece. The living room and dining room looked out over Twin Peaks. Upstairs was a room and bathroom, and it looked out over the city and the Golden Gate Bridge. On foggy days, we were often above the fog and you could see Mt. Tamalpais and the tips of the Golden Gate Bridge sticking out above it.

Neurology residency is a three-year training program after internship. The first-year residents examined all the patients admitted that day and wrote the notes and the orders for the patients' diet, activity, medications, blood and other tests. We followed our patients through the hospitalization – examining them daily, checking tests, evaluating and treating fevers or other complications. Once we had a tentative diagnosis, we could start to arrange discharge to home, rehab or nursing home. First-year residents were on call every fourth night, which meant we spent 36 hours in the hospital at one time and rarely got any sleep. Every first-year resident was supervised by a more senior second- or third-year resident. The senior resident knew all the patients well and had examined and written brief notes on them. Second-year residents had more time on rotations learning neuropathology, neuroradiology, electromyography and electroencephalography. The third-year residents 'ran' the inpatient services at Moffitt, the Veterans Health Administration Hospital (VA) and San Francisco General Hospitals. Each inpatient service had an assigned 'attending' – a neurology faculty member who met us at 10 a.m. every day of the week and reviewed all the patients we had admitted. We all examined the patient together.

This case-by-case learning was really an apprenticeship for future neurologists. We were taught how to assess what was normal or abnormal in a patient's gait, strength, coordination, sensation and cognitive function. We learned how to determine what part of the brain was malfunctioning based on the neurological exam.

The more cases we saw, the more we learned about what was normal and what wasn't. For instance, there is quite a variation in 'normal' gait or walk. Some people are pigeon-toed, toe-walkers whose butts stick out. Others are duck-footed and flat-footed with their buns tucked in. These variations are usually totally fine. The same with strength. Just because a tiny, skinny person isn't as strong as you or a muscle-bound type, doesn't mean the person has pathologic weakness. I learned to watch the posture, the swing of the limbs, the width of the stance, the speed of finger-tapping and the accuracy of touching the nose with the eyes closed. I began to see everybody in a new light. The postman coming up the walk, passersby on the sidewalk or in the parks – the whole world is a laboratory for evaluating disorderly movements.

I remember my first night on call as a neurology resident. I was in the San Francisco General Hospital emergency room – 'the Pit'. The ER was an amazing world! Unlike the Hopkins ER, people didn't usually walk in with knives stuck in the back of their heads or profusely bleeding from bullets that had hit them just around the corner. On the other hand, the place was always popping. The hospital is in the Mission District down near the San Francisco Bay. Ambulances brought in all the gunshots, attempted suicides and car/motorcycle accidents. All the drug overdoses. All the drunks, all the homeless, all the people who didn't have any other place to go. There were the male and female holding wards, each with about 15 stretchers for those who might or might not come into the hospital. There was the padded holding room for the psychotic violent cases. There was a tub room for delousing people who had been living in unhealthy conditions. There was a medical walk-in clinic across the hall. And of course, there were the trauma rooms.

There were always cases for the neurologist in the Pit. Found on floor (FOF), found on street (FOS) were the most common 'presenting complaints' on the chart upon arriving at the hospital. No history, no family. I got used to calling the operator and saying I needed the phone numbers of bars and houses near the site of the emergency. You could always count on the fact that when an ambulance arrived in a neighborhood, *somebody* noticed.

Many times, it was possible to learn what happened to the patient before the ambulance arrived by talking to what were called 'observers on the scene'.

So, as to be expected, my first night on call was a busy one. All of a sudden, I had gone from a simple intern to The Neurologist. I was completely ignorant, but the senior medical resident and the senior surgery resident somehow decided that I had some secret knowledge by virtue of the title on my name tag – Neurology Resident. We were all still in training but most of the medicine and surgical residents were ignorant about neurology and felt uncomfortable with the patients' odd behaviors. By about 10 p.m., I had already admitted a couple of people who had had strokes to Ward 42 (the neurology ward). Along with the nurses, I was responsible for their care. Five men in the male ward of the ER were in the midst of convulsions and I was responsible for stopping their seizures. They were being infused with intravenous Dilantin, a potent antiseizure drug. I went from one seizing guy to the next, pushing little boluses of Dilantin and then checking their pulse to make sure that I wasn't stopping their heart with the drug.

A medical resident came in and said, "You better come into the female ward and see this woman. She's 19 years old and two weeks postpartum, and her blood pressure is off the wall, and she is acting really weird." I left the guys – none of them were actively seizing anymore – and went into the female ward. A young woman was sitting up on a gurney, awake, but not making much sense when she talked, and she was writhing involuntarily on her right side. Her face was contorted, and her right arm was lifted up and twisting around. Her blood pressure *was* off the wall high. She was sick but this was weird! I had no idea. Acute onset of trouble speaking, headache and right-sided writhing movements.

I called Jack. "What the hell could be going on? What should I do?"

110

Of course, Jack knew the answer: "Hypertensive bleed into the left putamen. Get the blood pressure down. Get a skull x-ray to see if the pineal gland is shifted. Don't tap her. Call the neuroradiologists and take her up for an angiogram!" The pineal gland is about a one-centimeter structure right in the middle of the brain. It is often calcified and therefore can show up on x-ray. If a mass in the brain shifts it to the side, then the pineal won't be in the midline. This patient's pineal wasn't calcified and so an angiogram was indicated. I didn't think to call the attending because in those days it was considered a mark of weakness (not required the way it is today) to call for advice.

Whoa. This was certainly going to fill up my night. I'd have to be with her, and I'd have to pop up and down to check on my guys recovering from their seizures and my patients on Ward 42.

Within a few minutes, the woman was losing it. She rapidly became less responsive. The movements stopped, and she became paralyzed on her right side. We intubated her and hyperventilated her and gave her mannitol to shrink the brain. She temporarily improved. The neuroradiologist set up the angiogram to look at her blood vessels.

"Are you sure she really needs this?" the radiologist asked.

"What the hell else can we do? She's going down the tubes and maybe the surgeons can evacuate the clot."

She was completely unresponsive by the time we got her up to the angiography suite. Both her toes went up – a reflex that indicates evidence that the brain is under pressure. Bad news. Halfway through the angiogram she developed abnormal posturing of the two sides of her body (decorticating on the left side and decerebrating on the right side) – both clear signs that the pressure on the brain was getting worse. Really bad news. The angiogram showed a huge mass completely distorting the left brain and squishing the right side of the brain and pushing everything down toward the brainstem. Damn. She was dead. Or at least almost. For all practical purposes. And in a few hours, she really was dead. I never even got to admit her. Frankly even if we had known sooner, it was not something we could have fixed.

As an intern, I became familiar with death and losing my patients. During training, when I cared for people from the emergency room and didn't know them well, I could take their deaths in stride. Later in my career, I found the death of my patients very painful because I had often cared for them for many years and knew them well.

During training, I also learned that many people harbor diseases you cannot see. On the street, instead of seeing healthy people, I began to view everyone as having some unseen disease. I distanced myself from strangers. I also walled myself off from death. I saw so much of it; I couldn't survive if I let myself get too wrapped up in it. Instead of crying, I tried to think about how I could improve each patient's care.

That night was the first time I had to go down to the ER waiting room and tell a family that their loved one had died. I tried to explain what had happened as matter-of-factly and clearly as I could so the family could understand what had happened. "We did all we could but her very high blood pressure popped a blood vessel in the brain, and we couldn't stop it. The blood formed a huge clot and put enormous pressure on the brain. The brain is stuck in the skull and there is no room for the clot *and* the brain. The clot was too big and too deep to take out. Her left brain was badly damaged, the part of the brain that is crucial for talking and using the right side of the body." I paused to let this all sink in. Then I tried to offer some comfort. "Even if she had stopped bleeding she would have been paralyzed on the right side and probably wouldn't be able to talk. In a way, it may be better that she died rather than be so disabled. I am so sorry. I can at least assure you that except for the initial headache she wasn't in any pain, and she died peacefully."

The night wasn't over. I was called to see an intoxicated man who was found on the street, unconscious. I went to look at him. He had a big bump on the right side of his head, but a skull x-ray showed there was no fracture. He groaned if you pinched his Achilles tendon on each side but his right side moved better than the left. Both toes went up. His pupils were both small, regular and reactive. This was good because it meant his brainstem was still intact. Tickling his nose with a Q-tip (one of the least noxious ways to stimulate a semi-conscious person), he moved his right hand up to grab me, but the left hand and arm moved up toward his chest and his left leg stiffened – decorticating – indicating the cortex but not the brainstem was under pressure. Probably not a stroke or paralysis after a seizure – could be a subdural, a blood clot between the skull and the brain. I looked at the skull x-ray and the pineal gland wasn't calcified – so it didn't show up. (Back in those days there was no CAT scanner and certainly no MRI. It was a skull x-ray and/or angiogram. There were also 'nuclear medicine brain scans,' which weren't too great, and you couldn't get them emergently.)

I called Jack again. "The guy's obtunded, barely conscious, but hasn't blown a pupil. He is decorticating on the left, he's got this bump on his head, and he has no pineal gland visible." A blown pupil – dilated pupil – is a sign of increased pressure on the brain.

"Well, come on, Anne, this is when you want to catch them before anything bad happens. Call the neurosurgeons and get an angiogram and watch the pupil – if it starts to blow, give him mannitol. Intubate him now, so you can hyperventilate him also if you need to."

"Okay. Thanks, Jack. I don't think I would survive without your help. That other woman died, but you were right she had this huge putaminal hemorrhage!"

"Okay, okay . . . get to the new guy and let me get back to sleep!"

Up we went to the angiography suite again. The guy did start to blow his right pupil, but we hyperventilated him, and it went down again. He had a large right-sided subdural hematoma (a clot between the skull and the brain) and the neurosurgeons took him to the operating room and drained it. Cured. Back to the bars and the street. It was so sad that the social systems didn't exist to help him.

I checked on all my seizing guys and two had already woken up and left the ER. The other three were waking up and would be gone soon. All of them had alcohol or drug disorders with known seizures who had stopped their medicines. My two stroke patients upstairs on the ward had not had any issues and hopefully would improve on their own over the ensuing weeks.

So, I survived the first night! I had done my best and figured this job was challenging and tragic but exciting.

We rotated at Moffitt (the University) Hospital, the VA and San Francisco General Hospital. I liked the rotations at the General the most. The most amazing things happened there, and I learned things about human beings I never thought were possible. People drank all sorts of nasty stuff either to kill themselves or sometimes by accident. People drank Drano, rubbing alcohol and hairspray. People ate rat poison and washed their hair with pesticides. They shot up and snorted every drug possible and the intravenous drug users cherished their veins and never told you where the good ones were. The neurology cases were on Ward 42. It was an open coed ward, and the patient beds were arranged in rows facing the nurses' station. In the front row, nearest the nurses' station, were those needing intensive care – mostly comatose patients on primitive respirators. Next, after the intensive cases, came those who were breathing on their own but who were not cognitively intact – mostly patients suffering from head trauma, stroke and paralysis. Then the dementia cases, and then the patients with neuromuscular diseases. The demented old men were constantly crawling in bed with the other women. It was all so fascinating to see the various ways neurological diseases could affect people's lives.

Every fourth night, I covered the hospital, including the ER. One night, a guy from Grand Rapids, Michigan came in after having a cardiac arrest on the street. The doctors shocked him, and his heart started up again. I was called because the doctors were concerned about how damaged his brain might be from the heart attack. After a short time, he was awake, moving all limbs and somewhat confused. I asked him the year (it was 1975) and he said 1972. He said the president was Richard Nixon. I corrected him and said it was 1975 and that Gerald Ford was president. He laughed derisively. "Gerald Ford?! I went to high school with him. He's an idiot. Oh my God!" Wow. Great reaction. Acute Wernicke's (recent memory loss). I waited 10 minutes and asked him the same questions. Again, I got the first response virtually verbatim.

I brought around all the medicine and surgical house staff, and everybody was able to view the same response again and again and have a good laugh – not at him but at the response. Fortunately, the patient got better the next day and was discharged later, nearly normal. He didn't remember his initial response and all the repeats.

San Quentin, the California high security prison, always sent its cases to the Mission for evaluation, and one day I was asked to see a prisoner for a complaint of arm weakness. I walked into the male ward where the man was sitting on a gurney. He was huge and shackled with chains. Two prison guards were with him. He told me he had been in San Quentin for 20 years for murder and that he weight-lifted as a diversion. His biceps were bigger than my waist and his thighs were huge. He said that he normally was able to bench-press 400 pounds, but recently his right arm seemed weak, and he felt a pain down from his neck over his right deltoid and biceps when he tried to press the 400 pounds. I started to do my muscle exam to see if there was any weakness. When I got to the upper extremities, which was the key part of the exam based on his complaints, I was stymied by the man's extraordinary strength. I couldn't budge his deltoid or biceps. I tried hanging on his arm to see if I could elicit weakness, but he picked me up with no problem. I think I could have stood on his arm without it moving. His story was very convincing, however, and I didn't suspect him of feeding me a fake complaint as some patients were prone to do.

I called Roger Simon, who was my senior resident. Roger wore army combat boots, was 5'11" and weighed about 135 pounds dripping wet. Nevertheless, he loved to be the tough guy and get into the thick of things. He was always available to look over my cases and help if something peculiar came into the Mission ER. When Roger arrived, he asked the patient to hold out his flexed arm. He grasped the forearm and then put both feet on the wall and tugged. Hmmm. It did seem a bit weak. We asked him to hold his elbow out at 90 degrees and we both hung on it, bouncing up and down. Together we must have weighed almost 250 pounds. On the left side the arm didn't budge but on the right it did. Roger was convinced it was weak, and we ordered an electromyogram (EMG). It proved abnormal in just the distribution that Roger had predicted, and the man went to surgery to have a slipped C5 disc repaired. This man taught me to listen carefully to the patient's story, and if it fits the anatomy, investigate it. Don't just assume somebody is playing the system for some secondary gain.

We had a clinic at the General where the downtrodden, the poor and the homeless came to get their medications for seizures and other miscellaneous problems. Usually this was all pretty routine, but one afternoon, I picked up the chart of a woman named Blenda. She had a history of seizures and head injuries and had come to get her medications renewed. In the waiting room, I saw a pudgy, coarse-looking woman wearing old, tattered, wool clothing. When I called her in and asked her to get up on the examining table, I saw she had the apple-shaped body and skinny legs of a person with alcohol disorder. Multiple teeth were missing, and her hands were red and puffy. The palms of her hands were flushed. She tried to step onto the stool and then sit on the gurney, but she had to push hard on her knees to get up. That's interesting, I thought. She's pretty weak. I did the routine history and seizure exam and then I examined her muscles. She was very weak in both her legs and arms. I called in my attending, and we decided to admit her for the work-up of muscle weakness, what's called myopathy.

Once Blenda was on the ward, I came to take a more detailed history. She drank about a fifth of hard liquor a day – basically all she could get, and she said she didn't eat much because she spent her welfare check on booze. She lived on the street or in homeless shelters. I asked her where she was from and if she had gone to school. She said she grew up in suburban Detroit and went to Vassar. No way, I thought. She's got to be kidding. I told her I had gone to Vassar too, and I started asking her questions. She knew the names of all the Vassar dormitories and many of the professors. I asked her how she had come to be in such dire straits. She said that after college she had gone back to Detroit to be a television talk show host. Her program was called "Meet Blenda," and she worked there for several years until her program had been taken off the air. She came from a rich Michigan family, and she had been a debutante. After losing the show (mostly because of alcohol abuse), she went to California and over time became consumed by alcohol disorder until she was just another drunk on the streets. Ultimately, we found out that her myopathy was due to side effects of alcohol. She declined going to rehab. Social services were largely unavailable at the time.

She returned to the streets and the sad story stuck with me. So little difference between me and her. She was a debutante. She went to Vassar College. I certainly liked to drink. Could I succumb to it? Could I be beaten up by addiction the way Blenda had?

One evening in the Mission, I was called to see a young man who had been brought into the emergency room comatose and febrile. His girlfriend was with him and said that earlier in the day he had complained of a severe headache and stiff neck. Over the course of hours, he had become unresponsive, and finally, they had brought him to the ER. I set about examining him. He groaned to pain in all extremities and could move his limbs appropriately. His neck was very stiff. I looked at his two hands. They were very different. The right hand was robust and appropriately callused, but the other was delicate and smooth. There was no difference in size, however. When I asked his girlfriend, she said that he was very right-handed and mostly kept his left hand in his pocket. She said he had always been clumsy and had never played sports. I was stumped, but the first thing I had to do was make sure he didn't have meningitis. His symptoms – a fever high enough to suggest infection, a very stiff neck indicating irritated membranes around the brain and the fact that he was unconscious – were all consistent with meningitis.

I was worried about the left hand, however. Why was one side abnormal but not the other? Could he have a mass in his brain? I got a skull x-ray to see if the pineal was displaced but it turned out not to be calcified. I looked at the film myself and found nothing obviously wrong, so I set up to do the spinal tap. The nurse and I rolled him on his side. I cleaned off the skin of the lower back, numbed the area superficially with some lidocaine between two vertebrae and took out the four-inch needle. I inserted it slowly right between the two vertebrae taking out the stylet running down the center of the needle periodically to check for fluid. I felt a slight pop suggesting I might be in the spinal space. I removed the stylet again. The fluid came running out under very high pressure. I was scared by how high the pressure was. I quickly put the stylet back in to stop the flow while I got ready to actually measure the pressure on a gauge.

A healthy brain is surrounded by fluid and under no real pressure. When a person has an infection, the volume of the fluid increases and compresses the brain. There is only so much space in the skull and the increased pressure causes altered consciousness. A tumor can also compress the brain by taking up space in the skull. That was why the patient's high spinal fluid pressure was so alarming. Taking out fluid at the spinal level though might 'suck' the brain down thereby putting pressure on the brainstem where all the vital fibers travel. The fluid was cloudy, and I assumed it was meningitis and started him on antibiotics while I went off to examine the fluid. I found no bugs (otherwise known as bacteria!). I was terrified that my spinal tap had made him worse, so I watched him like a hawk all night.

The next morning, I was called by the radiology attending who wanted to know about the patient. He said his skull x-ray was very interesting and called us down to look at it. A small tooth-like structure and what appeared to be a small bone were visible right along the bone above the left ear. He said it must be a 'teratoma' – basically an embryonic tumor that develops in the womb from a twin that doesn't separate to form a whole embryo. Basically, this guy had been living for decades with his twin in his head. Well, not exactly an entire twin. More like traces of what could have become a twin.

We did an angiogram and the entire cerebellum, a structure at the base of the brain controlling coordination, was occupied by this tumor. That definitely explained the clumsy hand. A damaged cerebellum made the hand hard to control. When the neurosurgeons took out the tumor, they found hair, teeth and bones. Apparently on the day he was admitted, the tumor had ruptured and leaked noxious fluid into the spinal fluid–filled chambers of the brain (ventricles) causing what's called a 'chemical' meningitis. I was amazed that the guy lived and hadn't died from the spinal tap, but it taught me that as long as you anticipate a worst-case scenario and act accordingly, you can tap almost anything.

One Sunday morning, Jack and I were driving to Lake Merced for our weekend run when we saw a car parked by the curb and a small crowd of people on the sidewalk attending to someone lying down. We pulled over and got out. Dressed in shabby shorts and T-shirts, we pushed our way through the crowd. An older woman was face-up, flat on the sidewalk, her arms and legs straightening spasmodically. Someone was trying to stuff a piece of cloth into her mouth.

"Hey. We're doctors. Can you tell us what happened?"

The people looked at us suspiciously. A man came over and said he saw the woman pull over. She looked distressed and so he asked if he could help. She had told him she couldn't see and asked him to get her a drink of water. He went next door to ask for water and when he came back she was lying on the front seat having what appeared to be a convulsion. He had just now pulled her onto the sidewalk.

"Have you called an ambulance?" Jack asked. We could see this was no convulsion.

"Someone is off calling one now," the man said. We knelt down by the woman. She had a pulse and was breathing but she was unconscious. We took the cloth out of her mouth and watched her. Her breathing was rapid but regular, and she looked well oxygenated. We pulled up her eyelids; her eyes were looking straight ahead, but every couple of seconds they bounced down, stayed for a second and bounced back up. Her pupils were so tiny, you could barely see them – even when you blocked out the light. This was bad news, very bad news. We both knew that these findings were most consistent with a hemorrhage into the pons (in the brainstem) – a critical area of the brain about the size of a nickel through which most of the information passing to and from the brain must pass. Usually, it occurs in people with hypertension and is fatal.

We asked the people if the woman had a purse. Now the crowd was even more suspicious of us. I found it in the front seat and opened it up. I found her name and address, and even more remarkable, I found a prescription for an antihypertensive medication with a doctor's name on it. We were near a pay phone. Jack stayed with the woman and began to write up a history and neurological examination on borrowed paper.

I called the doctor's answering service and miraculously he called back. "Yes. I know Mrs. So-and-so. She has hypertension but otherwise is pretty healthy. I always find her BP high, and she rarely takes her medication."

Wow. I came back to tell Jack. The ambulance had arrived. We put the new information from the doctor (including his name and address) into the note. We referred to ourselves as "observers on the scene" and we chronicled the grim sequence of events, gave a differential diagnosis and addressed it to the neurology resident on call. Later we learned that the poor woman died several hours later in the hospital. Unfortunately, nothing can save these hemorrhages even nowadays.

The story, however, became the tale of the neurology service for a while. Most patients were brought in 'found on floor' or 'found on street,' so to get this whole detailed sequence from 'observers on the scene' was really amazing. It was equally amazing when the case was presented at brain cutting several weeks later, and one of the faculty said suspiciously: "Who are these 'observers on the scene'?" When he learned Jack and I were the 'observers,' he was impressed with the job we did.

I loved neurology. I had had trouble taking care of general medicine patients. They weren't very interesting to me. The medicine patients were primarily distinguished by laboratory numbers rather than by direct examination. In contrast, in neurology, I felt totally different. The patient with neurologic problems was a person I could observe, examine physically, understand, diagnose and try to help feel better.

Jack and I made quite a team. Jack read voraciously. I skipped around the journals and read selected abstracts. Generally, Jack had read the articles I had an interest in, and he could summarize them for me. We both were fascinated by movement disorder patients, but we had almost no experience with these patients because they were usually outpatients not hospitalized inpatients. Parkinson's disease, Huntington's disease, tremor, dystonia and tics. Our dinners and evenings were spent discussing some aspect of neurology or some other science. We always subscribed to the *New England Journal of Medicine*, *Neurology*, *Annals of Neurology*, *Science*, *Scientific American*, *Natural History* and *National Geographic* at home. We got the newspaper every day. Usually, I grabbed the front page while Jack read the rest of the paper including the funnies. Then I read the funnies and he looked at the front page.

One day when we were sitting around reading the newspaper, Jack brought up the subject of children. I told him, not for the first time, that I didn't particularly want children. It was way too much work, worry and responsibility. I wasn't sure I had the energy for parenting in addition to the energy needed to be a scientist, clinician and teacher.

Jack said: "Oh come on. Children will be so fun, and I'll personally promise to help with everything."

"I've only had one babysitting job in my life, it was disastrously scary, and I was completely incompetent. Furthermore, I have no mothering instinct."

He kept bringing it up, and we discussed all the possibilities. He pointed out that we could hire a live-in babysitter. To me all his plans made sense. He convinced me that he would help and it would be wonderful. I had seen how naturally Jack played with his niece and nephew. I knew him as a devoted man. I decided that if there was anyone I could raise children with while maintaining my career it was Jack.

So, at the end of my first year of neurology residency, we decided to start 'practicing.' After all, most people don't just get pregnant at the first try. Furthermore, I had an IUD – the famous Dalkon Shield – and likely, my uterus wouldn't be receptive to an embryo for several rounds. We wanted to have the baby at the end of my second year when I had scheduled elective time. Jack was going to be finishing residency, so he wouldn't be on call that first year.

Well, son-of-a-bitch! The machinery worked well, and I was pregnant a month after the Dalkon Shield was removed. I figured it out when we were up at Walter Henze's wedding in Seattle. I remember being completely elated and telling everybody that it had worked. I felt high. Hypomanic. I couldn't sleep but I was awake and happy.

I told my mother. Her first reaction was "Oh, no! You know that no male Young ever lived to see a grandchild. They all died too young. I hope your father survives this." Wow. Instead of congratulating me, my mother thinks I have killed my father by becoming pregnant. We told Jack's parents and they were thrilled. The only problem was that Jack's mother appeared to have developed systemic lupus erythematosus. She was fairly ill and we were in California, on the other side of the country.

Morning sickness wasn't a big problem, and I was working hard during the entire pregnancy with regular night calls. I had to run the inpatient services at the San Francisco General, Moffitt and the VA. Then I was slated for two months of pediatric neurology before my four months of elective. The baby was due in the middle of my pediatric neurology rotation. Several times during the pregnancy, I got colds and couldn't take night call, so Jack filled in and took extra nights. He was a year ahead of me in residency so there was no problem with him helping me out. Unfortunately, his mother became very ill about eight weeks before the baby was due. Her 'lupus' turned out to be a deadly lymphoma. She died and I felt like I had lost a mother. She was such a welcoming, supportive and interactive woman and I knew she would have been a fantastic grandmother.

Candace called. She had heard the news and was calling to offer a key piece of advice: "Hire a full-time, live-in nanny. Take it from me, it's the only thing to do. It's worth all the money it takes. Even if you have to spend one of your salaries on it. Hire the person now before the baby is born so you'll be all set." Candace had become a mother at age 19 and yet had somehow managed to work extremely hard at the lab and complete the requirements for her graduate degree. She had a live-in nanny. If she could be a scientist and a parent, so could I.

Jack and I talked about it. We'd discussed the possibility before getting pregnant and now it made sense. As residents, we had all sorts of weird, unpredictable schedules. Having someone live-in gave our schedules a lot of flexibility. Our house had a 'room down' (a room behind the garage in many San Francisco homes) that could easily be a little apartment and we could fix it up with a bed, table, refrigerator, sink and stove. It even had its own bathroom and a separate entrance. It was perfect.

We placed our first ad and got many responses. We interviewed several but most were either too expensive or psychology majors who were mostly interested in *studying* a newborn. Then Joan called.

Joan got to the 'interview' late, running up the street after missing the bus. She was 19 and told us she "needed a job real bad." She hadn't graduated from high school and was the second youngest of seven children, but she said she had plenty of experience babysitting and could give us references. No child psychology, no ambitions. Just needed a job. We went back and forth on the choice. Joan was energetic but a high school dropout?

Maybe she'd really screw up. Nevertheless, she was affordable and we decided to hire her.

Waiting for the baby was really annoying. "When are you going to have that baby?" Everybody asked. Everybody had advice. About everything.

All the cases on pediatric neurology were 'basket cases'. Tiny heads, blank looks, weird seizures, terminal illnesses. It was so sad to see and yet I was eight months pregnant and about to have *my* baby. I could only envisage a tragedy with it. We were picking out names. Girls were no problem. We wanted a girl to be named Jessica Pero Penney after Jack's maternal grandmother, Jessie Pero. Jessica was the 'in' girls' name and it was also a 'family' name. Boys' names were much harder. I thought Cyclops was good based on all the disasters I was seeing clinically on pediatric neurology.

I had a 'continuity of care' clinic on Wednesday afternoon, and I had 14 patient follow-up visits scheduled. Seizures, headaches, post-stroke care. I was nauseous and felt terrible. I was afraid I'd throw up on the patients. I made it through and went straight home to bed. That was when I realized I was having contractions. When Jack came home, he made me some dinner but I couldn't eat. He felt the contractions too and called the obstetrician. The contractions were 30 minutes apart, and the doctor said call him back when they were closer together. We went to bed and around midnight I rolled over. Liquid rushed out. I just peed all over the bed! I shifted and another whoosh came out. The bed was wet. I leaned down to smell it. Babies! It didn't smell like urine at all. It smelled just like Johnson & Johnson baby powder! I nudged Jack. I think I'm leaking amniotic fluid, smell this. He sniffed. We called the OB again and he told us to go to the hospital.

The baby didn't seem to want to come out. I was doing all the Lamaze breathing stuff, but even after a couple hours I still wasn't dilating. They put me on a Pitocin drip that essentially gave me one giant contraction with little stronger ones on top of it. After 16 hours, the doppler monitor started registering type II decelerations of the baby's pulse which we knew forebode anoxic brain injury or cerebral palsy. Jack and I said to hell with this natural birth Lamaze thing, we want the baby out. Now. By C-section. The doctors agreed. I opted for general anesthesia, and the baby was out – she had had the umbilical cord wrapped around her neck. Good thing we did the C-section.

Jessie was a tiny 5 pounds, 15 ounces, post mature and wrinkled, but she had her thumb in her mouth, and she had all her fingers and toes. Jack was ecstatic. I started breastfeeding, and Jack practiced changing diapers. I came home after five days. Joan moved in. She ate hamburgers, French fries, fried chicken, butter and whole milk. Vegetables were foreign to her. But she was good with the baby. Jessie was either sleeping or laughing and attentive. With all of us, she had postprandial colic but otherwise she was fine, and Joan didn't have any complaints.

I only took two weeks off total. I actually found it completely boring looking after the little autonomic machine. It was fine in short doses. Babies are very noisy – grunting, burping, puking, pooping, crying, cooing. Jessie slept in a crib next to our bed. I was lucky to be able to breastfeed her when I got home. Several times during the night I woke up to nurse her again. At work I used a pump, but I only saved the milk a couple of times. It was difficult to find a place to actually pump since no private spots were available except a stall in the bathroom and there was no place afterwards to refrigerate it. So, Jessie had formula during the day and me at night. Of course, that meant that 'sleeping through the night' was not an option. I told Jack that if I was going to do this, he had to change her after I fed her. Jack became the Master Changer. I got Jessie from the crib, and she cuddled in and nursed. Then I nudged Jack and passed the baby to him, and he changed her in a flash and had her back in the crib sleeping soundly. I swear he could do it in his sleep. He liked to bathe her and feed her, too.

I, on the other hand, was entirely incompetent. The first day I went back to work, I instructed Joan how to make up the formula. "Oh, it's easy," I said. "You just mix one part formula with one part warm water."

Later in the day, Joan called me and said that Jessie was throwing up the formula. She thought maybe I had the dilution wrong and it was too thick. The truth was revealed. The MD/PhD pharmacologist was a complete ignoramus. It should have been one part formula to two parts water. Shortly thereafter, I was clipping Jessie's nails and I clipped off a chunk of her thumb.

Then there was the diaper fiasco. We had decided to go natural and get a cloth diaper service. Every Monday they picked up the dirty diapers and dropped off a batch of clean ones. Joan didn't particularly like the stinking mess of dirty diapers but in general there were enough clean ones to double-diaper her through the week. Using only a single diaper was risky as they were thin and didn't hold all of the urine and poop. Then Jessie got her first bout of bad diarrhea. We were going through the diapers quickly. By Saturday, we had to use a single diaper each change or we'd never make it to Monday. Jack was downstairs doing the laundry and I was changing Jessie. Off with the diaper, wipe, wipe, wipe with the Wet-One, powder, slip the clean one under, grab a wad of diaper on each side and slip in the safety pin. There. A heart stopping, ear splitting, pathetic scream suddenly emanated from Jessie. Holy cow! What's going on? I tugged at the diaper. One side didn't move. My heart was pounding, my blood pressure dropping. The screaming continued. I pulled back the other side of the diaper. I'd pinned Jessie to the diaper! I was going to faint. I screamed for Jack. Hands on Jessie, holding my head down between my arms.

Jack came bounding up the stairs. "What's going on?"

"I've fucking pinned Jessie to the diaper!"

Jack told me to lie down before I fainted. He unclipped the safety pin and slipped it out. Minor injury. Jessie stopped crying and looked content. I was a wreck. I felt completely incompetent as a mother and questioned my decision to have her.

Jack was laughing. "You're worse off than she is. It's no big deal, she's going to be fine."

For the first six months or so, I measured Jessie's head circumference every day. Her head was on the big side. I was paranoid. I envisioned the worst. Hydrocephalus. A neuroblastoma or medulloblastoma. Jack said it was nonsense. He had a big head too. Not to worry.

As Jessie developed in a few months into a little human being with a unique personality, I realized how much I loved her. We spent all our free time with her. We walked everywhere with Jessie. First in the Snugli and then in the Gerry pack. We shifted carrying time between the two of us. Golden Gate Park. Stinson Beach. Mt. Tamalpais. Ocean beach. Up and down over the hills. We went to Yosemite when she was just four or five months old and walked all over the valley. We took her to the lakes in the Oakland Hills to play in the sand and water. We took her to the Society for Neuroscience meeting.

We took her to our friends Walter and Sarah's house in Tonasket, Washington. Sarah was pregnant and I had Jessie on my back when we went on an eight-kilometer cross-country ski race. Going down one hill, there was a low hanging branch and I ducked but Jessie was conked on the head. Oh my God. Was she hurt? She was so special to me but thankfully she was fine. When we reached the finish line, Jack and Walter were already there.

Jack said a man had come in just before us and said as he crossed the line: "At least I beat the pregnant woman and the woman with the kid on her back." We all had a good laugh.

I was chosen to be chief resident in my third year. Normally, this is a special honor. In my case, however, it wasn't quite as prestigious. We started residency with six residents in our year. One was pediatric neurology. There would have been five adult residents second year but one dropped out and one had already done two years of neurology research, so he jumped to third year. That left three of us. Then for the third year, one of them said he was going to leave halfway through the third year to do his elective time as a stroke fellow at Massachusetts General Hospital. Then there were two ... and the other one wasn't exactly a 'people person'. I got the job.

Jack was doing a fellowship in neuropathology at the VA. He rode his bike down from 10th & Pacheco, across the Golden Gate Park and over to the VA. I walked or took the car. We began looking for jobs. We wanted to stay in San Francisco but there was no space or resources – only closet-sized laboratories and very limited start-up funds. We looked at Cleveland, Ohio; Rochester, New York; and Ann Arbor, Michigan. I had written a draft of a grant to study thyroid and dopamine receptors. I prepared a presentation that I could use to give talks. On visits for job interviews, we couldn't take Jessie. That's what stopped my nine months of breastfeeding for once and for all. On a visit to Ann Arbor, Jack awoke to find me rummaging under the bed for Jessie. I had dreamt she was with us and had fallen under the bed.

Ann Arbor was great and Sid Gilman, the new head of the neurology department at the University of Michigan, offered me a job as an assistant professor and Jack another year of fellowship in neuroanatomy followed by an assistant professorship the next year. Fully equipped labs and start-up funds for us both. It was the best deal, and we signed on. Because of Sid's interest in motor disorders, I wrote a whole new grant to study glycine and GABA receptors in spasticity. Sid helped enormously with the grant, and I submitted it in two different forms to the National Institutes of Health (NIH) and also to smaller foundations such as the Easter Seals Society, the United Cerebral Palsy Foundation and the March of Dimes. Once a grant is submitted, of course, you have to wait months to hear the result. Jack's fellowship in neuroanatomy with Sarah Newman was all set. He would learn the latest anatomic methods to examine specific pathways in the brain.

In medical school, Jack had worked in neurovirology, studying progressive multifocal leukoencephalopathy, for which he'd received the Weil Award as a medical student (quite a feat). As a postdoctoral fellow, he studied a mouse model of polio. He liked the work but mostly he liked the anatomy and studying things under the light and electron microscope. He was concerned that the breakthroughs in neurovirology were going to be on the molecular and not anatomic level. We found ourselves talking a lot about the motor system. Maybe we could determine the neurotransmitters of important pathways in the motor system. We decided that his expertise in neuroanatomy would complement my knowledge of neurochemistry. Together we would make a great team. We were both excited to begin our joint research.

I had seen several people with Parkinson's disease during my training and found taking care of them and their medications, like L-Dopa, challenging and rewarding. I had also seen one man with Huntington's disease – an inherited disorder causing slowly progressive involuntary movements, poor balance and loss of cognition. Because of my PhD with Sol, I knew a lot about the drugs and pathways that could be affected in these diseases.

The real estate boom in San Francisco meant that we sold our house for more than double what we had paid for it. We, therefore, had to buy a nice house in Ann Arbor or pay capital gains taxes. We chose a house that had a bedroom distant from the rest of the house for a live-in babysitter so everyone could have some privacy. We asked Joan if she would at least come with us temporarily to give us time to look for another babysitter. She agreed; she'd never left San Francisco and saw it as an adventure. We planned a route by way of Portland, Oregon to see my old friend Les and through Tonasket, Washington to see Walter and Sarah. We hired movers and packed everything up. We headed up the coast.

When Jack, Jessie, Joan and I arrived at Les' new place, it was midday and very hot.

By now she had moved off the commune with a new girlfriend. We pulled up in the driveway and got out. Les was standing on the fence of the pigpen at the end of the driveway throwing stuff from a big cardboard box into the pen. She waved and we walked over introducing Joan and little Jessie who was one and a half. She explained that she and her girlfriend had a new business; they didn't raise the rabbits or sell their feces as the commune did. They had a building, which provided space to butcher, skin and package the rabbits. There was also a room with freezers where the meat was stored before it was sold to grocers. There was a holding room where the rabbits were housed before they were killed. Rabbits were supplied by various people, many of whom were sick of their pet rabbits at home. Les said she'd be done in a second. She was just chucking rotten rabbit meat to the pig. She said it was a bummer that the freezer had failed and a whole lot of meat had rotted.

When she finished, she got down, wiped her hands and gave us big hugs. She took us into the house and introduced her new girlfriend, Kathy, who was sitting at the kitchen table drinking beer and smoking a cigarette. The table was littered with empty beer bottles and ashtrays full of cigarette butts. She introduced their foster daughter who was about 11. The place was a dump, and I could see that Joan was looking around and obviously wondering what she had gotten into.

The next morning, I sat down with Les. I noticed that her teeth were badly decayed.

"Why don't you see a dentist?"

"I don't have any dental or health insurance and we're losing money, and we can't afford to cover Kathy's medical costs for her bad back or my dental care."

I said, "What are you doing? Why are you trying to run this business if it's losing money?"

She said, "It's such a cool business and it will soon be making money."

In addition to taking care of the rabbits, Les was also working full-time at the sawmill. Kathy was not working, supposedly because of her bad back. I asked Les, "How much is the mortgage, the utilities, the feed for the rabbits before they are killed, the processing and packaging materials, the living expenses? And how much do you get per rabbit or per pound of meat and the furs?"

"Hmmm ... I don't know. I've never made that calculation."

"Let's do it now." We added up the costs and the profits and it was clear without looking at the details that it was a losing operation. Even with her salary from the sawmill! I said, "Les. You have to dump this thing. You're just getting yourself into a hole. At least your girlfriend should get a job. I'll help you if I can, but you have to get a life!"

I was really depressed when we left and so was Jack. Les had been my best friend growing up and Jack liked her a lot too, but her life seemed so sad. She was no longer the ambitious and talented basketball player with whom I'd collaborated or the articulate person organizing civil rights marches. Somehow, she now had no anchor to help stabilize her life. Although she was trying to make ends meet, she wasn't practical or realistic about how to go about it. I worried about how her future would go and I wished I could help.

We went on to Walter's house. Here he was! In family practice in Tonasket, Washington. He and Sarah were hand building a stunning house at the eastern edge of the Cascades. While building, they were living in a small frame house with wood stoves for heat and cooking. He and one or two other family practitioners took care of all the people in a 50-square-mile area just south of the Canadian border. The odd thing was that just over the border in Canada there was substantial tourism, game parks, dude ranches and agriculture. On the US side, it was an impoverished apple-growing county with a lot of people on welfare and in need of a family doctor. They should thank their lucky stars for Walter. He was so smart, so patient and so caring. He once had a girl brought into the little four-room hospital that he ran who had had a serious head injury. Walter immediately diagnosed an epidural hematoma – normally a terminal event unless taken care of emergently – just on the basis of what his clinical astuteness allowed him to observe. He took the girl to the operating room and called a neurosurgeon in Seattle who coached him through an operation to stop the bleeding and remove the epidural. A plane then took her to Seattle, and although the girl rebled on the way, she survived to be a healthy kid. There are few doctors I would entrust my health to but Walter was definitely one of them.

We spent a great couple of days with Walter, Sarah and their new daughter, Talia, before heading out for Ann Arbor via a stopover at my parents' house. On the far side of the Black Hills, our clutch went out. It was the Fourth of July weekend, and we were driving a Peugeot diesel we'd named Eeyore. In that rural part of the Midwest no one would fix it on a holiday weekend. I knew how to drive without a clutch – another thing my father taught me, so we just continued on. I changed gears by revving and pausing at the right time. On the way across Minnesota, we got into some spectacular thunderstorms that scared Joan but which I thought were wonderful. California did not have thunderstorms, but I had grown up with them, and I thought they were scary but exhilarating! Going through traffic in Chicago without a clutch was a challenge but we made it to my parents' house in Winnetka. Joan was feeling more comfortable by this time and was reassured to see their fabulous house on Lake Michigan. When I was in college, they had moved from Snake Hill to a lot on the lake where they'd built their own house.

Jack and I went to an auto parts store on the weekend, and they instructed us on how to check and redo the clutch. The two of us messed around for an afternoon, but eventually we got it fixed. It wasn't that hard. Maybe if we failed in neurology, we could become car mechanics.

We spent the weekend at my parents' house on the lake, and they enjoyed playing with Jessie. Then we were on our way to Ann Arbor. Wildflowers bloomed in the median strip of the highway. The house was empty when we arrived, and that first night we slept on the floor. The moving van arrived and our stuff from San Francisco was unloaded. All the leaves had fallen off our potted jade trees but miraculously they later grew back. The night-blooming cereus made it too, which we took as a positive omen for our new place and this next step in our careers.

8

• • • • •

Setting Up Our Labs
and Clinic

We soon felt at home in Ann Arbor, a midsized, liberal town with a strong student presence that was like an oasis among the rural cornfields of the Midwest. The university was large, and the University Hospital and Veterans Health Administration Hospital served as local and referral hospitals for much of the state and northern Ohio. The neuroscience building, where our laboratories were located, was two blocks from the hospital. Our house was four miles west of our labs and on the edge of farm fields. With no sidewalks or paths near the road, only one neighbor next to us and a few houses behind us through the woods, we were fairly isolated. We loved being 'in the country'.

As a new faculty member, I was given a 'start-up package' to give me support for the first two years of laboratory work. Once the start-up package was spent out, I was expected to get my own grants to support my salary and all the lab activities. Since running a laboratory was like managing a little business, I had to plan how to get the most monetary support possible. In the United States, the National Institutes of Health (NIH) offered the best source of

135

support in the form of grants. By then I was well aware that applications had three yearly deadlines for submission. Many hundreds of grants were submitted at each deadline from faculty all over the country. Grants were then reviewed by committees of some 30 peer scientists from other institutions. The reviews took about four months. Each grant was expected to request several hundred thousand dollars of support for each year's expenses and to cover a period of three to five years. In addition to the NIH, nongovernmental foundations in the country give out smaller grants of $10,000 to $35,000 for one year only. These organizations each had their own Scientific Advisory Boards and the reviews were completed more quickly than the government ones.

I decided to get a head start and write several grants while I was still a neurology resident in San Francisco. I worked on them in any 'free' time I had during night call. I wrote several applications and submitted them before I even got to Michigan. My grant proposed to study glycine and GABA receptors in paralyzed animals with spasticity and I submitted to several nongovernmental organizations. Soon after I got to Michigan, I learned that both the Easter Seal Foundation and the United Cerebral Palsy Foundation had approved my grant, but the March of Dimes had rejected it. I was able, with Sid's coaching, to keep them both.

I had submitted the same proposal to the National Institute of Neurological Disorders and Stroke (NINDS), which is part of the NIH, for both an early career grant covering my salary and another version to cover lab, personnel and animal costs. My Teacher Investigator Development Award was approved by the government to cover my salary for five years. It would begin in five months. My other grant to the NINDS – a so-called R01 – had fared less well with a priority score of about 220 (on a scale of 100 to 500 – 100 being the best). The relatively high score meant that I would get no funding for the grant and I would have to rewrite

136

and resubmit several months later a revised grant that could be funded in a year at the earliest.

Sid suggested I call the health science administrator (HSA) at NINDS for my grant and ask him/her if he/she could give me any information or advice. He said that frequently the HSAs sat in on the grant reviews and could provide the investigator with some tips about the reviewers' concerns and how to rewrite it.

I looked at the postcard I had received from NINDS that indicated that my HSA was a woman named Nancy Wexler. I told Sid that I hated calling people in the first place and in this case it seemed like cheating to call up to get inside information about my grant.

"Nonsense! That's their job. Their raison d'être. Everybody does it," said Sid.

I built up my courage and called. Ms. Wexler answered the phone. I introduced myself and told her the grant number, title and that I was assuming it wouldn't be funded but maybe she could help me with advice. "Hold on a minute," she said. "Let me look it up."

I waited. She sounded friendlier than I'd imagined.

"Weelll. Actually, this is a very interesting grant," she said. "In fact, it addresses issues very important for paralyzed veterans and others. There is almost no research going on in this area and yet spinal cord injury is such an important public health problem. Ordinarily, your grant would not be funded this time, but our program people discussed it and we think we should fund it. It will have to be 'specialed' and we won't know until after Council meets but I think you will probably get the grant."

"Wow!! Really?" I was excited.

"Yes. Congratulations!"

Yahoo! I couldn't believe it! Four out of the five versions of the grant I submitted were funded, and the cool thing was that I was going to be able to keep them all! Between the grants and my start-up-package from the university my salary would be funded for five years and my laboratory for three years. I couldn't believe my luck.

We would now be able to spend 80 percent of our time in the laboratory and 20 percent of our time seeing patients (one day a week). This schedule allowed a lot of time for our basic research each week and then one day a week we would see patients. We were lucky that Sid supported this allocation of time. Many department chairs would require young faculty to do more clinical work – reducing possible efforts in the lab.

Having received the grants, Jack and I decided we could have another kid. We had discussed it. I had been paranoid about struggling for grants. Now things had solidified funding-wise. Joan had also decided to stay as she liked Ann Arbor. She had nothing really to look forward to in San Francisco. She learned to drive a car, and we bought her an old used Ford to drive the kids around in. She tried taking some courses at the Y but she wasn't interested in any further education. She became friends with various plumbers and painters that came to do odd jobs on the house. We paid her a good salary, paid her social security and bought her health insurance.

Soon enough the experiments I'd proposed in my grant turned out to be complete failures. My hypothesis had been that the severing of an animal's spinal cord and resulting paralysis would cause changes in glycine and GABA neurotransmission below the level of the injury. If there were changes, perhaps we could find better drugs to relieve spasticity. These experiments might help people who had become paralyzed, including a large number of veterans. The idea was sound but carrying out the experiment on rats was horrible. We had to sever the animal's spinal cord, which of course meant their legs became totally paralyzed and numb. The animals treated their legs as if they were not their own body and started to chew them off. I had to paint their legs with nasty tasting picric acid to prevent their self-destruction. Their bladders also became unable to empty by themselves, so I had to pinch their bladders to empty them three times a day.

As in graduate school, I didn't want to go to the lab in the middle of the night to squeeze rat bladders. So ... I brought the cages of paralyzed rats home and put them on our bathroom counter. Jessie couldn't understand why there were rat cages in our bathroom. Not only were these experiments difficult to carry out but the data also didn't clearly show any differences in glycine and GABA neurotransmission between the spinal cord above and below the cut. I did my best to do all the experiments I had proposed in the grant, but it was frustrating. Once I'd collected enough data to disprove my hypothesis, I decided that it was not worth pursuing further.

Instead, Jack and I decided to use our time to study the main pathways of the motor system. For neurologists, the most important pathway was the corticospinal tract – the nerves that go from the surface of the brain all the way down to the spinal cord. The corticospinal tract was critically important for controlling movement and was affected in strokes and brain tumors. We could use the same approach I had taken in graduate school looking for the neurotransmitter of the granule cells in cerebellum. Our approach was not as elegant as for the cerebellum because we could not selectively kill only the nerve cells of the corticospinal tract. With brain surgery, though, we could remove the part of the brain where the corticospinal tract begins.

Jack and I made a good team doing these experiments. Jack did the surgery and made and evaluated the lesions and I conducted the biochemical experiments. We examined rats and, in collaboration with Sid Gilman and colleagues, we also examined cats and monkeys. Unlike the spinal cord work, these experiments produced unequivocal evidence in rats, cats and monkeys that glutamate is the neurotransmitter of the corticospinal tract. This was a big deal. In neurology, this pathway is affected in many disorders and now we knew how we could evaluate this glutamate pathway in illnesses. We published our work in several papers in neurology and neuroscience journals.

We suggested to Sid that we start a Movement Disorders Clinic. We hoped to focus on Parkinson's disease, Huntington's disease and related disorders. Movement disorders fascinated both of us and we liked the notion that it was a subspecialty relying on direct patient observation. During graduate school, Sol's lab did many studies of drugs affecting the part of the brain called the striatum, which has the highest dopamine concentration in the brain and is abnormal in Parkinson's and Huntington's. I was comfortable with all the medications used in the treatment of these disorders because many were studied in Sol's lab. Even though we hadn't trained in movement disorders, we were excited about starting a clinic and figured that we would soon learn. It wouldn't have been possible to open a specialty clinic without having specific training had we been in a major medical area like New York or Boston, but in Michigan, there were no other clinics that specialized in movement disorders. In no time our clinic was filled with interesting patients. Jack loved being a doctor and interacting closely with his patients. During my clinical training, I, too, had learned how rewarding it was to have long-term relationships with patients. The Movement Disorders Clinic met one day a week. In the morning, Jack and I would each see our private patients and then, in the afternoon, we would supervise and teach residents and fellows evaluating those with disorderly movements.

We were soon learning by our own mistakes. At least we could discuss the cases at home together and try to figure things out. Essentially, each of our patients had two neurologists. On weekends, we watched videotapes of movement disorder patients sitting in a chair, walking and performing other parts of the neurological exam. We continued our habit of taking long walks together during which we discussed patients and potential lab experiments to figure out more about how movements are controlled. We would often stop to draw circuits in the dirt or sand as a platform for discussing new experiments.

Another factor that contributed to our thriving Movement Disorders Clinic was that the Michigan neurologist who had taken care of all the families with Huntington's disease in the area moved to the Mayo Clinic less than a year after we arrived. We told Sid that we were interested in taking over the care of the Huntington's families in our clinic. Although Jack and I saw all comers, we sort of split our practice. Jack saw the 'hypokinetic' disorders – Parkinson's, progressive supranuclear palsy and multiple system atrophy – and I saw the 'hyperkinetic' disorders – Huntington's, Tourette's, tremors, dystonia. It fit our own personalities. Jack was calm and measured with a wry sense of humor who approached problems linearly whereas I was more scattered, active and nonlinear.

Huntington's disease is a heart-rending illness. It is inherited as a dominant gene, which means it is carried from one generation to another and does not skip a generation. Each child of an affected parent has a 50 percent chance of inheriting the gene. It usually begins in a person's mid-thirties, well into a woman's childbearing years, but it can begin as early as two or as late as ninety. In the 1950s, the geneticists at Michigan had done a thorough study of the epidemiology of HD in Michigan and Minnesota. We had access to the multigenerational family trees they had put together for many families who received their medical care at the university.

The disease begins insidiously with little jerk-like movements of the limbs or body or with personality changes. People lose weight. Gradually, coordination is affected, and the movements become pronounced. With this, individuals start to lose their ability to do any complex tasks. Speech becomes difficult to understand, and choking is nearly universal. Eventually, individuals become unable to communicate, and they writhe in their beds when disturbed. Death usually comes from infections such as pneumonia when patients can no longer clear their throat secretions, have difficulty swallowing and inadvertently inhale tiny pieces of food. The time from the beginning of the disease to death is on average 15 years but for some it is shorter and for others as long as 30 years. Depression, irritability and apathy are common. Occasionally, patients are psychotic. Many of the mood changes are treatable with medications. There is no cure, so care revolves around maximizing quality of life for both the patient and his/her family.

In contrast, Parkinson's is likely multiple diseases and is not usually inherited. It usually begins in a person's sixties (although there is quite an age range). It begins insidiously with stiffness and slowness of movement and possibly a shaking tremor. Fortunately, it is treatable with medications that function as so-called 'dopaminergic agents'. These agents are probably *the* success story in neurology. They replenish the dopamine pathway that is diminished in Parkinson's disease. As I learned in medical school, when a patient who is stooped and virtually immobile is given a pill, within half an hour they can walk normally. Managing the medications, however, is an art. You can get quite a bit from books or journals, but only with experience is it possible to figure out the best strategies for treating each patient. With good therapy, people with PD can live to a normal age, although their quality of life certainly declines considerably at the end. Unfortunately, the treatments do not stop the underlying disease process. Eventually, the patients get many complications from the medication and progressive disease. They die most frequently of infection such as pneumonia – again because the patients can't clear their secretions and often inhale pieces of food that can lead to disease.

With each person, we became their principal care doctor, managing their day-to-day problems and trying to maximize productive and satisfying lives. We also treated the spouses and family members and tried to give the best advice about surviving a family member's illness. For Huntington's disease, of course, genetic counseling was important for family members so that they could make informed decisions about career and childbearing. This subspecialty of neurology was just what we wanted. We were motivated by the lasting relationships we could form with patients and their families and hoped the patients would inspire experiments we could pursue in the lab. We were excited about the many faceted challenges and rewards running the movement clinic could bring.

At home, we were settling in. We rode our bikes the four miles to work. We equipped our house with a wood stove and a solar system for heating the hot water. We ordered cords of wood and spent crisp, cool afternoons splitting wood. I used to imagine each piece of wood as the head of a person or an idea that I hated and then whap! It split into pieces; it was very gratifying. It's a great way to release anger and aggression – much healthier than either holding it in or lashing out at a person. We heated our house for 10 years with wood. We were early adopters of solar power, managing to heat our water with solar for 13 years.

A year after we got to Michigan, I got a phone call from my old friend Les Moore. I hadn't heard from her since visiting her in Oregon and I was too busy to worry about whether or not she'd been able to improve her situation. Now I learned that things had only become worse. She told me she needed money and that she was 'on the lam' from the law because she had taken someone else's two-year-old child who was being abused. She said the child had suffered terribly and she had to get him away from his biological mother. I wanted to help but I had to tell her I couldn't give money, because if my support was ever discovered, I would lose my medical license.

Overall, we were content in Ann Arbor. We could live in the country and yet be near town. Jessie was becoming her own little person in ways that often surprised me. One time when she was three, we went to a park. Another little girl just Jessie's size was on the swing and a small tricycle was on the grass nearby. When Jessie walked over to the tricycle and sat on it, the little girl jumped off the swing, ran over and slugged Jessie in the face, knocking her to the ground. I ran over to Jessie, picked her up and told her what my father would have told me. "Run over and slug that girl back as hard as you can!" Jessie froze and looked up at me. "Mom! You don't fight them with fists. You fight them with words." I couldn't believe my ears. Of course, she's right, I realized. What kind of mom am I?

Then came the time when Jack and I had to take the board examinations for certification in neurology and psychiatry. Both psychiatrists and neurologists were 'boarded' by the same organization. The first part, written boards, was to be taken a year after residency and the second part, the oral boards, a year later. The oral boards for neurologists required in-person examinations of both a neurology and a psychiatric patient. Jack was ahead of me and passed the written boards without a hitch – he could have passed *any* multiple-choice test. The next year, I took the written boards too and actually did better than I had on most of my previous multiple-choice tests. We decided to sign up for the oral boards at the same time, and we were arbitrarily assigned to take the test in Milwaukee, Wisconsin. We were lucky to have Joan to watch Jessie overnight while we were away. Needless to say, we were nervous. The oral board exams were intentionally difficult, and you couldn't really prepare for them. The most difficult part was the live examination of a psychiatric patient; the psychiatrists were known to flunk 50 percent of the applicants.

The neurology part of the boards was tolerable but we both failed the oral psychiatry exam. It was the first examination that either of us had failed. Jack's patient was very quiet and answered his questions in one or two words. Only 20 minutes was allowed for the patient exam, and so at the end of the time, Jack knew almost nothing about the patient and therefore couldn't discuss much with the examiners.

My patient was a homely, slightly obese young woman with coarse features, thin dirty blonde hair and pimples. My description may be unkind but the truth is I usually saw strangers in a very matter-of-fact way. I did not always see them favorably. Nevertheless, I was professional as I calmly asked about her problems. My patient professed to have basically everything wrong with her. She said she was from a dysfunctional family with drug and alcohol problems and also said she was a depressed, abused, suicidal, paranoid, hallucinating young woman. She had 'spells' for which she was admitted to the hospital. I asked about the 'spells' and from her description they sounded as if they could be temporal lobe seizures. Goldmine for the neurologist!

My exam over, the psychiatrists began asking me questions. They asked if I would have treated the patient for temporal lobe seizures and whether I would have put her on Dilantin as the doctors at the hospital had. Dilantin is often prescribed for seizure disorders but has side effects causing thickening of the ridge over the eyes, a swarthy complexion and thickened gums. In my typical blunt, direct and seemingly uncaring way, I replied, "No, she's already ugly enough, and Dilantin will just make her uglier. I'd put her on carbamazepine or phenobarbital. They should be at least as effective and don't have those side effects."

The exam ended abruptly. I had flunked. Even though I was just trying to keep the woman from getting even coarser features as a drug side effect of the Dilantin, the shrinks couldn't abide by my 'already ugly enough' statement. My evaluation said that I was too blunt, unsympathetic and impulsive in my comments and I should have been more understanding.

We both had to take the oral psychiatry part of the boards again, and this time we were assigned to San Francisco. Again, Joan took care of Jessie. My patient was a piece of cake. He gave his whole history logically and coherently, and all I had to do was listen. Jack was not so lucky. The patient he was originally assigned refused to participate at the last second, and they couldn't find a suitable replacement except for a patient who refused to say a single word. Jack flunked again. Finally, on the third try, Jack got a patient who gave a history and he passed. Jack and I never completely got over the humiliation of failing this exam. A few years after we took the exam, this oral in-person psychiatry part of the neurology boards was discontinued and instead candidates were tested on a video vignette of a patient.

We might not have much control over the evaluation criteria for our professional certification, but when it came to hiring people for our lab, we made all the rules. We interviewed undergraduate, graduate, postdoctoral and MD/PhD students who were interested in working in our labs. Some students just wanted a brief lab experience, but several MD/PhD candidates wanted to earn their PhDs in my lab. I knew from my experience at Hopkins that pursuing both degrees requires hard work and dedication. I tried to accept applicants who exhibited a true passion for science. I have a high bar when it comes to such a qualification. The Nobel Prize–winning neuroscientist Rita Levi-Montalcini was to me the epitome of the passionate scientist. As a Jew in Italy during World War II, she was not allowed at the university and had to hide to avoid capture but was so passionate about science that she didn't let the situation defeat her. Instead, she set up a lab in her bedroom at home and subsequently in the basement. She and her family survived under false identities and after the war came to the US where she taught and continued her research at Washington University in St. Louis. Levi-Montalcini was an inspiration and I wanted to train people whose passion for science approached hers.

Once an applicant became a student in our labs, each one was given a project to work on. To develop their intellectual independence, we also encouraged them to formulate independent

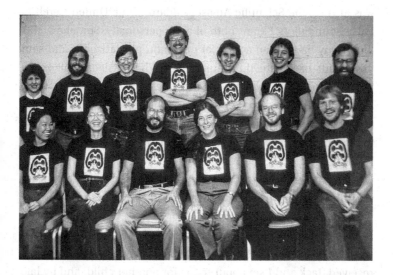

Figure 8.1 The lab about 1985.

We are all wearing an image of a glutamate receptor autoradiogram by Tim Greenamyre. Back row, left to right: Dorene Markel, Simon Starosta-Rubenstein, Zane Hollingsworth, Daryl (surname unknown), Eric Richfield, Jim Olson, Roger Albin. Front row, left to right: Dorothy Chu, Helen Pan, Jack, me, Timothy Greenamyre and Brian Ciliax.

hypotheses and experiments. Each student usually became the first author on at least one published manuscript describing their work. Equally important, they became part of our lab family (Figure 8.1). We had frequent parties at our house where we all played, ate and drank. Every year, we made a new lab T-shirt that we all wore on the same day at the annual meeting of the Society for Neuroscience.

Shortly after setting up my lab, Sid asked me to review a grant that had been submitted to the United Cerebral Palsy Foundation. He was a member of the foundation's Scientific Advisory Board. I read the grant and, lo and behold, the grant was almost identical to the grant that I had submitted a year before. The grant was written by a junior faculty member at Hopkins and his supervisor was also on the Scientific Advisory Board of the United Cerebral Palsy Foundation. I knew both of them personally. Somehow, this junior guy had gotten a copy of my grant, plagiarized it and sent 'his' grant back into the Foundation. What a sleazeball! I told Sid and he agreed it was clearly unethical behavior. I wrote a critical review and voted not to fund the grant. I didn't mention the plagiarism in my review. In the future, however, when I had many opportunities to review this person's grants and papers, I was not a friendly reviewer. What really dismayed me, though, was that somebody had actually copied portions of someone else's work! It was a harsh reality test then, and as I have since learned, this behavior is not uncommon.

Jack and I realized how much we loved Jessie and what fun it would be to expand the family. Encouraged by the grants I'd already received, Jack and I set about trying for another child, and by late January 1979, I was pregnant. As with Jessie, the pregnancy did not particularly slow me down. Jack and I were working on applications for additional grants with Sid. We applied for an additional federal grant with the idea of acquiring two grants for our experiments. The more funding we could get, the more experiments we could do. We were asked to join a group putting together a proposal for a large program project grant to support positron emission tomography (PET) scanning of the brain, a technique that was then relatively new. The University of Michigan had a Nuclear Medicine Division that was renowned for its development and application of diagnostic procedures using radioisotopes to label tumors, thyroids, hearts and brains, and we wanted to collaborate with the head of the division to set up a center where we could use the new radioisotope procedure to image the brain.

The CAT scan, which had only been around since the mid-1970s, took a picture of the brain by exposing the brain to x-rays at different angles and then using a computer to reconstruct the data and give detailed pictures of the *structure* of the brain. It was a great scan to look for blood, tumors or pus. It couldn't assess brain *function* though. A PET scan used a short-lived radioactive substance that gave off x-rays, or positrons. The radioactive substance was given to the patient intravenously or by inhalation, after which it enters the brain and then gives off x-rays (radioactive decay) that are measured by computed tomography. One could measure various metabolic activities (not just structure) by this method. The technique could look beyond structure to *function*. Specifically, we wanted to use the PET scan to test the ability to measure the brain's receptor distribution in disease.

As I knew well, drugs and neurotransmitters interact with other cells via receptors. We wanted to try to label GABA, opiate, dopamine and acetylcholine receptors in postmortem brains using receptor autoradiography and then figure out how to apply the method to PET scanning in humans. If we could do that, we'd be able to measure all sorts of interactions in the brain.

Our laboratories were a floor below a laboratory studying how the brain utilizes sugar by using $[^{14}C]$-labeled glucose in animals. They injected the $[^{14}C]$-glucose intravenously, then killed the animals and measured the uptake of the glucose in various brain regions by exposing brain sections to $[^{14}C]$-sensitive x-ray film. Although this method showed both the amount and localization of sugar utilization, we couldn't use the $[^{14}C]$-sensitive film for neurotransmitter receptors, which were measured using tritium $[^{3}H]$ – a much weaker radioactive label. Was there a way we could use a similar strategy to measure neurotransmitter receptors? Earlier that year, a new x-ray film sensitive to tritium $[^{3}H]$ – the radioactive isotope we used to label receptors – became available. We developed a new method of measuring receptors in sections of the brain using this film. The method measured the number of receptors in clearly defined anatomical brain areas. We proposed to measure neurotransmitter receptors in postmortem brains from people who had died with Huntington's, Parkinson's and

Alzheimer's diseases. We would thus be able to discern how an illness affected the specific circuits in the brain.

We needed to hire a lab manager to oversee our equipment, supplies, budgets and students. Zane Hollingsworth came to interview. He had a master's degree in toxicology. "What are your aims in life?" I asked. "I want to manage a laboratory," he said. Perfect. His career goal is to have *this* job. We hired him and he was soon a key component of the lab. He was very organized and detailed. He had a quiet, wry sense of humor, and he had a deep knowledge of Ann Arbor's incredible resources.

We started to collect brains from people dying of neurologic and non-neurologic diseases, building our brain bank. Our friend, Ira Shoulson, at Rochester, New York, already had a brain bank and agreed to collaborate with us. In addition, we'd proposed to study the ability to measure neurotransmitter receptors in rats, as models of human disease. These animal studies would show us whether the methods we proposed to do in humans would work.

Our project also proposed to study brain glucose metabolism in Huntington's disease patients. Work from UCLA researchers had shown that even before the brain shrank in the disease, its ability to take up radioactive glucose was reduced. PET scanning might therefore become a way of identifying early disease and might serve as a marker for when treatment should be started even prior to the onset of symptoms. We proposed to scan groups of brothers and sisters who had a parent with Huntington's disease yearly for five years and gather blood samples to be used for DNA analysis later on. Each participant had a PET scan, MRI scan, neuropsychological testing and a videotaped neurological examination. As part of the study, we also asked for funding for a genetic counselor and a nurse. Human studies are much more complex than animal studies. The equipment was unreliable. The subjects were unreliable. The investigators were unreliable. In short, it was no trivial project to scan people over years in a prospective study to try to determine the first changes in the brain that occurred in Huntington's disease. The concept was great, yet in modern society, people move, investigators move, equipment changes and the ability to actually get measurements of chemicals in the brain that can be compared over time is challenging. It impressed upon me the difficulty of doing studies in humans.

The whole grant was written, assembled and submitted for the June 1st deadline. The NIH wrote back and said that the grant would be reviewed at the University of Michigan Medical School by an outside team of expert scientists on September 26, 1979. Sid and the other project leaders ran multiple practice reviews throughout the summer to hone our presentations. By August, I was seven months pregnant and really uncomfortable, but as September approached and the weather cooled, I felt better. Because I had had a C-section with Jessie, I was scheduled for an elective C-section for this baby – on October 10. First the site visit review, then the baby.

Mid-September, the weekend before the site visit, Jack and I were grocery shopping, as we usually did during the Michigan football game. It was the best time for shopping since the stores were empty – everyone was at the game. Jack and I had made the mistake of not opting for season football tickets when we'd first arrived in Ann Arbor. All new faculty were offered the option, but after that if we didn't sign up, we couldn't get season tickets later on. Later, we regretted the decision because we could always sell the tickets for a profit, and our seats would have become better each year. Michigan had the biggest college football stadium in the country, and at games it was always full.

As we were shopping, I told Jack that I felt really terrible. I felt nauseous and my back hurt. He said, "I know one other time when you felt like this – when you were in labor with Jessie. Do you think you are having contractions?"

We stopped in the aisle. Sure enough! I was having contractions. We bought the groceries and went home and called the doctor. He said to lie down and see if they went away. But they persisted and even came more frequently. We called again and this time he asked me to come to the hospital. The two of us drove in, leaving Jessie with Joan. They checked my blood pressure and urine. I had ketones in my urine, and the nurse accused me of not eating properly. I told her I was eating very well – three meals a day. She looked askance at me and put in an IV. She said that they would see if hydration stopped the contractions. They proceeded to put three liters of fluid into my system! Three liters of room temperature liquid pumped directly into your circulation cools you down tremendously. I started to shiver uncontrollably. Jack found some blankets. The contractions weren't stopping, so at midnight, the doctors said they were going to do a C-section. Do you want general anesthesia or an epidural? Jack and I discussed it. With Jessie, I had been exhausted from all the time in labor and so general anesthesia seemed the best. This time, though, an epidural sounded best. We asked if an attending physician (not a resident) could put in the catheter. It was only September and the residents likely hadn't done many procedures. An attending physician and a resident arrived, anesthetized my back and stuck in a big needle. It didn't hurt a bit. Even though I had done hundreds of spinal taps as a resident, this was my first time experiencing one. Either it really was an innocuous procedure or my own endorphin levels were killing the pain. They injected the anesthetic into my spinal space. First my feet went numb, and then after several minutes, my abdomen was numb. Then it moved right up to my armpits – higher than it should be. The inside of my arms was numb and so were the fourth and fifth fingers of my hands. I knew that if the anesthetic moved higher, I would stop breathing. I said I was a neurologist and hoped they had an AMBU bag ready (a mechanical bag to breathe for a person).

I told them again that I thought the level was too high, and the doctors said, "Nonsense!" Why were they just ignoring my pleas? Did they doubt my knowledge? Only when I insisted did they take out a pin and stick it in my chest, arms and fingers to check that I was indeed numb. Surprised and somewhat appalled that I was right, they tilted me up. They had screwed up and had removed the catheter so they couldn't remove any anesthetic. At least they had an AMBU bag.

Fortunately, I was fine and the numbness from the anesthetic went no further but I noted that again the medical system was more than fallible. I wondered what happened to patients who didn't have my expertise.

The C-section was incredibly quick. Jack was there watching and comforting me. Within no time a little baby girl was at my side. We named her after my grandmother, Elsie – Ellen Buckingham Penney. The anesthetic wore off slowly. When I was finally able to get up, my muscles worked but my legs were still numb, and I had no idea of where my legs were. I had to look at them or else they might go their own way. I staggered with Jack down to my room. The next day, I was back to normal, and I realized I could work while Ellen slept. I reviewed some papers and edited a manuscript I was preparing to submit for publication.

The site visit was happening in two days! I practiced my presentation in bed. I wanted to know the material cold and make no mistakes. The day of the site visit, I got up from my bed, put on a dress and went down to the conference center to give my presentation. The visiting reviewers were all male and very polite. I was given a stool to sit on while I presented. I doubt they had ever seen a woman present a project, especially three days postpartum. After finishing and answering questions, I went back upstairs and was discharged home from the hospital.

At home, I waited by the phone to answer any of the site visitors' questions. The phone call came with many detailed questions, which I answered as best I could and then crossed my fingers. I hoped that my demonstration of commitment dispelled any reviewer's concern that I would be another woman who abandoned a career to care for the children. At least they knew I already had one child and a live-in nanny. Ultimately, we got a very good score, and our project in particular suffered no cuts. Jack and I now had a second federal grant funding us. Although I knew that I had done well in my presentation, I was pleased that my pregnancy/delivery had apparently brought sympathy and kindness from the reviewers.

Ellen turned yellow – jaundice. Her liver wasn't metabolizing a protein called bilirubin. High levels caused the skin to turn yellow. I had to take her in every day to have her bilirubin measured. It was high and they threatened to take her back into the hospital again. I worried about cerebral palsy because high bilirubin levels could damage the striatum – a critical area for motor control. Every day, I took her out into the yard to expose her to the sun because UV light was known to help clear the bilirubin. Gradually it worked, and she was able to stay at home. Unlike Jessie, Ellen only fell asleep in our arms. If I put her down sooner, she cried until I picked her up. If she went to sleep in our arms and then we put her down in her cold bed she woke up immediately. So, we found out that we could warm her bed with a small heating pad and then take it away just before we put her down. That worked perfectly. Ellen nursed for four months, but because I had to take several trips, my milk supply diminished and she eventually gave up and took the bottle. Jessie had immediately put her thumb in her mouth after she was born, and she never used a pacifier. Ellen, on the other hand, became pacifier dependent.

Shortly after Ellen was born, we all went off to the Society for Neuroscience meeting in Atlanta, Georgia. Joan, Jessie and Ellen came along. Joan took care of the kids in the evening and during the day. Jack or I put Ellen in the Snugli and carried her around the meeting. It was at that meeting that I first met Nancy Wexler. She had long blonde hair, was beautiful, vivacious and surrounded by all sorts of admirers. I thanked her for helping me with my grant.

9

• • • • •

Neuros in the Lagoon

The family members leading the local Huntington's disease chapter at the time – the Michigan Chapter of the Committee to Combat Huntington's Disease – made an appointment to see me on a Saturday morning. They were very concerned because their doctor of many years had left, and they wanted to meet me because I was taking over their care. They wanted to see if I was going to be a good doctor for the HD families. I met with them, answered all their questions and assured them I would do all I could to help.

Soon after, Nancy Wexler was scheduled to come to the university to give the weekly departmental neurology meeting called 'grand rounds.' I learned that Nancy was a graduate of the PhD program in clinical psychology at the University of Michigan. While in graduate school, her life was turned upside down when she learned that her mother had HD. She decided to write her thesis about the complex psychological, medical and social issues that arise when a person is at risk for HD – as she now was. In gathering data, Nancy had become friends with many of the Michigan HD families. She was a founding member of the

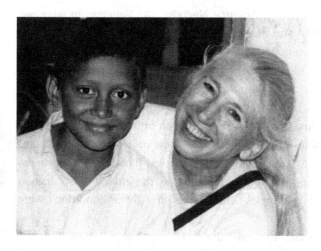

Figure 9.1 Nancy Wexler with a young Venezuelan child. Courtesy of Julie Porter.

Michigan Chapter of the Committee to Combat Huntington's Disease. As I found out later, the Chapter leaders had encouraged her to come to Michigan to check me out.

Nancy appeared with her flowing blonde hair, dressed in colorful but casual clothes and smelling of perfume. That was the first time I experienced the incredible presence that she brought with her wherever she went (Figure 9.1). With great conviction and excitement, she talked about a new strategy for approaching HD. She explained that prominent molecular geneticists, particularly David Housman at MIT, had suggested that the gene could be found using the new recombinant techniques if a large family with multiple affected generations could be found. The idea was to collect blood, skin and even semen samples from as many extended family members as we could and bring them back for the geneticists to study in their lab. In 1972, Nancy had heard of such a family in Venezuela at the symposium marking the 100-year anniversary of George Huntington's description of the disease.

She'd contacted Dr. Americo Negrette, the Venezuelan who had first observed and described the affected family and in 1979 had gone with two neurologists to investigate. She particularly wanted to study this big extended family since there appeared to exist large sibships who were the offspring of two parents with HD. If both parents had HD, it was possible that some offspring had two HD mutations instead of one – one mutation from *each* parent. Perhaps these 'double dose' people would show more severe or different symptoms. At grand rounds, she showed pictures of Venezuelan families living in houses on stilts in the middle of a lagoon surrounded by jungles. The houses and living conditions were very poor.

After the grand rounds, she and I went out to lunch. I'll never forget that lunch. She was the most compelling and stunning person I had ever met. I wondered how anyone could be at risk for HD and yet have such self-confidence, persistence and a mesmerizing, infectious character. I was immediately in awe of this extraordinary woman. How did she do this? How did she cope? How can immersing yourself in the problem actually help? When she spilled her iced tea at lunch, she looked at me in a way that seemed to wonder whether I was seeing this clumsiness as a first sign of the disease. I wasn't. But I *was* scrutinizing her carefully – something involuntary for a neurologist. I just wanted to know more about her and what made her tick. It was wonderful and terrible at the same time. She was at risk for HD, a veritable genetic Russian roulette. A 50 percent chance of getting the disease. All I wanted was to make that risk go away. I watched her, and I could tell she was self-conscious about her movements and dexterity. I hope she realized that I only wanted to help. The lunch was short though, and she left soon after. I felt a desire to learn more about her.

A few months later, I was invited to attend a workshop of the Hereditary Disease Foundation (HDF) in Los Angeles in early January 1980. A prominent neuroscientist, Eugene Roberts, was on the Board of the HDF and had suggested I attend. We had first met at Hopkins, when he site-visited Sol's laboratory to review a grant Sol had submitted. I had presented my work on [^{3}H]-strychnine binding to the glycine receptor. He had been impressed and even offered me a fellowship, but I had to decline since I was scheduled to do my clinical training. He kept up with my research interests, however, and talked to me routinely at the annual Society for Neuroscience meetings.

The HDF was founded by Milton Wexler, Nancy's father, in 1968, the year after Nancy's mother was diagnosed with HD. Milton was a prominent clinical psychoanalyst for many in the Hollywood arts community. He was motivated to find help for Nancy's mother and others suffering from HD and had been struck by how clandestine and unimaginative scientists can be. Meetings where scientists got up and gave a series of talks seemed to go nowhere fast and rarely led to new approaches or collaborations. He set up the HDF in a new way. The organization was dedicated to funding basic HD research grants and pilot projects that hoped to give the scientists enough preliminary data to apply for future federal funding. To drive the research forward more quickly, however, he also organized workshops that were modeled on the candor and interactive nature of group therapy sessions he was used to leading.

Workshop participants were chosen to include people from a wide range of scientific backgrounds – genetics, basic neurobiology, immunology, neurology, psychiatry, pharmacology and pathology. No one was allowed to give prepared talks or show slides. Rather, Nancy or Allan Tobin (a UCLA neuroscientist Milton hired to help organize and run the workshops) guided an open-ended discussion. I found the workshops incredibly stimulating and interesting. Sol had taught his students not to be afraid of showing one's ignorance by asking basic questions. I had no problem asking geneticists and others what their jargon actually meant. I also liked to speculate – to imagine possibilities and ask, What if? Thus, participation was great fun. Nancy was at the workshop, but I never got to talk to her since she was off with this person or that person organizing dinners and discussions. She was always working. She was clearly very knowledgeable about science as well as the personalities of the scientists and prominent donors. Dinners at the workshop were frequently at an artist's or movie star's house like Julie Andrews or Jennifer Jones. Once we had dinner at architect Frank Gehry's home. Unfortunately, since I never went to the movies, I didn't appreciate the extraordinary group of artists, writers and actors who attended as much as I should have – Frank Gehry, Peter Falk, Carol Burnett, Jack Lemmon, Sophia Loren, Carrie Fisher, and Walter Matthau. It was clear, however, that these stars found it fun to mix with the scientists and vice versa. Nancy floated between both groups, making everyone comfortable and enthusiastic.

In late January or early February of 1981, Nancy called me at home in Michigan from Washington, DC. She explained that she was organizing a trip to Maracaibo, Venezuela to pursue studies of the families that she had presented two years before at Michigan. Would I be willing to come down for a week and make a trip to Lagunetas, the stilt village on a lagoon off Lake Maracaibo that she had shown slides of at her Michigan talk? My job would be to examine the family in which two parents with HD had together birthed 14 children, all of whom were living. She explained that she was organizing several neurologists to participate for one to two weeks in March or April. I would be the only neurologist on this segment of the trip. After her description of the wilds of the Venezuelan jungle surrounding the village, I wondered if I could do it. I hated snakes, spiders and other critters. On the other hand, if Nancy, who always dressed beautifully and had the spontaneity, charisma and a rare grace in the way she cared for others and articulated her concerns, could function in the jungle, I supposed I could too.

I also realized instantly that this was a potential entrée into a series of field studies not unlike the sojourns through New Guinea and other remote spots that Richard Johnson had lectured to us about in medical school. I didn't want to let this opportunity go by, but I worried about leaving Ellen, who was only 18 months old and Jessie, who was four. I sat down with Jack. I asked his permission to leave him alone with the kids and go to a potentially dangerous place. It didn't take him long to say yes. He had seen enough HD and its consequences to realize the importance of a project aimed at finding the gene and a cure. He also acknowledged to me that his primary focus was Parkinson's disease whereas mine was Huntington's disease and therefore it made sense for me to participate. I could see more than a bit of his jealousy that I was getting to go off on this adventure and I hoped he could participate on any future trips.

What to wear? Certainly, the hiking clothes I had for the Rockies and Lake Superior were not appropriate. I had spent a summer in Arizona but never any time in the tropics. I decided to take long cotton pants and short-sleeved cotton shirts. Even in the jungle, with pockets and absorbent cloth, I should be okay. I packed my neurology tools, a straw hat, suntan lotion, tennis shoes, sandals, a bathing suit, my Swiss army knife, flashlight, a small thermometer and a little first aid kit.

Since Jack and I had been married, I had never gone out of the country without him, and I had never been to Central or South America (except Tijuana). I didn't know any Spanish, and I had no real idea of what I was getting into. Jack and the kids took me to the airport to see me off, and I hugged and kissed them goodbye. I flew to Miami. At that time, Pan Am flew directly from Miami to Maracaibo, Venezuela. We flew over Cuba, Jamaica and finally the coast of Venezuela. It was a clear night and there appeared to be a sizable city along the edge of the lake as we approached the airport but, elsewhere, there were very few lights dotting the flat countryside. I had a couple of drinks on the plane. I was nervous. I hadn't any real idea of what was ahead, and the people were basically unknown to me. The plane came down low, made a left turn and landed around toward the north (every flight I have taken there since has landed the same way). I muddled my way through customs and picked up my bags. In addition to the Venezuelans, the airport was filled with men wearing work clothes who were obviously there to work on oil rigs. Steve Uzzell, the photographer from the project who'd come to pick me up, had little trouble spotting me, the young neurologist from Michigan. He was tall, bearded and muscular. I was fairly tipsy. He drove us back to the hotel. Along the road, the odor of raw sewerage wafted through the windows. A fierce humid, hot wind was blowing.

During this initial trip, I learned a lot about myself and my relationship with Jack. I missed him terribly. Not only did he always handle the tickets, passports and transportation details but he was my soulmate; we constantly talked about science, the project at hand and people we encountered. He wasn't there, and I suddenly felt naked. The people on the team were all strangers to me, and I had little chance to talk to Nancy, who I barely knew, since she was extremely busy organizing the group, identifying patients and families, dealing with the Venezuelan collaborators and negotiating the political scene. The one person I did know was Ira Shoulson, the neurologist and HD expert with whom we'd collaborated on the brain bank. He had come down for the first couple of weeks and was overlapping with me for a day before he returned to the States.

The team stayed at the Hotel del Lago, a nice hotel on the shores of the lake in Maracaibo, Venezuela. Nancy reserved one large suite that we used as an office for group meetings and that held all the papers, labels, copiers, blood-drawing supplies, coffee, soft drinks and snacks. We met daily in the office at 7 a.m. and Nancy went over the plan for the day. Most days, the team drove a half hour to San Luis, a barrio on the lake south of Maracaibo where many HD families lived. They were fishermen who went out at night to get the best catch and then sold the fish at markets in Maracaibo. A government clinic existed in San Luis where a doctor and nurse worked two mornings a week to see people from the community. The rest of the time the clinic was empty.

Nancy's goal was to put together a detailed family tree of all the HD families, take blood and skin samples from each family member and examine each person neurologically and cognitively. The blood and skin samples would be sent back weekly with one of the team members to Jim Gusella's laboratory at Mass General. Jim had done his PhD with David Housman at MIT and was hired by Joe Martin, head of neurology at Mass General, to join his neurology department at Mass General. The blood was for DNA analysis and the skin was a source of cells that could be frozen and used for future experiments. We aimed to see and examine as many persons in the family tree as possible and trace the inheritance of the gene through several living generations. We had to be certain of diagnoses we made because any mistakes could mislead the geneticists. My job was to do neurological exams and sometimes take blood and skin samples. I viewed my role as a soldier in the army fighting HD and I followed orders from Nancy, La Jefa!

The second day in San Luis, I was on my own and Steve decided to work with me to photograph various patients as I examined them. The photographs too were to be part of the study. Steve set up his camera just outside the 'bee' room, so-called because the inner room connected to it had a huge beehive and bees were constantly intruding on our space. The room had an examining table opposite the door and the patient was brought in and lifted into a sitting position on the table. I began with the eye exam that I had practiced the day before with Ira and with Fidela Gomez, an Argentinian nurse, who taught me the Spanish phrases I needed to conduct the exam. Steve's camera was huge and heavy, and he was standing in the sun – the temperature was about 100 degrees in the sun and about 90 degrees in the room. It was humid and sweaty. I stood in front of the patient and started to do the exam.

"Anne. Could you step six inches to the left, please?"

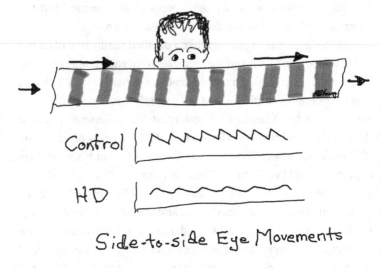

Figure 9.2 Cartoon of test of optokinetic nystagmus.

The striped tape moves right to left in front of the person and the eyes move quickly back and forth as the stripes go by. If I raised or lowered the tape too much the photographic shot would be ruined.

I took a large step to my left. I reached into my pocket and pulled out my optokinetic nystagmus (OKN) tape (Figure 9.2). The tape was a cloth strip with red and white vertical lines about one inch wide. The idea was to hold the tape about six to eight inches in front of the patients and ask them to look at the lines as I pulled the tape across their vision. Normally, the eyes jerk from line to line, looking from one to the next. (It's like the sensation you have when you look out the window of a train as all the trees are rushing by and you can feel your eyes jerking from side to side.) In Huntington's disease, the speed and amplitude of these eye jerks decline as the disease progresses. In advanced HD, the jerks have completely disappeared.

I drew the tape from right to left and then left to right. Again, Steve interrupted. "Anne, could you move the tape about a half an inch down because it is right in front of the eyes?"

I lowered the tape about four inches. The day went on like this – Steve constantly giving instructions for where I should stand and how I should move. I overreacted, thinking I was being more than accommodating.

That night, Steve and Nancy shut themselves up alone for some time. The next morning (the day before the trip to Lagunetas), Nancy came to my room and said point-blank that Steve couldn't work with me. He was insulted by my lack of attention to his instructions and indicated that I was just like all the other arrogant, narcissistic doctors he'd met who felt superior to photographers.

I was crushed and embarrassed. I thought I had been trying to be as accommodating as possible. Nancy said that Steve had decided not to go to Lagunetas and would likely return to the US. Now she wasn't sure if any of us should go. I had managed to screw up the whole trip. I couldn't believe what I had done. I explained that I respected Steve and had tried my best to follow his suggestions. I didn't have a clue as to what the issues were for Steve, but I was willing to apologize and try my best to do better. Nancy, Steve and I met, and I apologized for my mistakes. We talked and he proposed that I look through the camera to see what he was seeing; if we could manage to work together, he would reconsider going on the trip.

When I looked through his camera, I was able to see his perspective. When he was trying for a very close shot of the patient's face, the positioning of the tape made a big difference. Moving the tape down a half an inch allowed him to see the eyes moving as well as the tape. If the tape was moved down four inches, it was completely out of the picture and the movements of the eyes made no sense. Likewise, when I was six inches to the side of the patient, he could see both of us but if I stood a foot to the left, I was out of the picture. I learned to develop a sense of where the camera was in back of me and draw a line in my imagination that helped me move in such a way to accommodate the camera. Steve also learned to feel more comfortable telling me directly if I was in the way, and if he said move two inches, I did exactly that.

The upshot of all this was that Steve agreed to go on the trip to Lagunetas.

I took a blanket and pillow from the hotel and a backpack with a change of clothes, a clipboard, my neurology tools, my pocketknife and the small emergency aid kit I'd packed. The team consisted of about eight Americans and six Venezuelans.

We left Maracaibo at about 10 a.m. on the 50-foot Venezuelan Coast Guard boat that had been arranged for us through the US Embassy. With us was a fisherman from the HD family who lived in Lagunetas so that he could guide us into the right lagoon. The Coast Guard had no detailed maps of its own. The lake was very large – almost like an ocean. We went out beyond sight of land and passed many, many active and inactive oil wells on the way. Inactive wells were evident by the four 20-foot-tall cement corner posts protecting their well heads. The active wells were large, dark and dirty but had buildings on each where at least two dozen oil men ate and slept. We pulled up to one to refuel the boat. Despite the bright, relentless sun, the heat, sweat and grime on the rig made me feel we were traveling through Joseph Conrad's heart of darkness – the wicked colonialism.

We went further down the lake beyond the oil fields until we were again within the sight of land. The fisherman pointed toward a place on the coast. As we approached, we saw a small group of boats coming toward us. A gap appeared in the trees along the shore, and we noted that waves were breaking at the entrance. The crew started using poles to test the depth as we drew nearer the shore, and eventually, not far from the waves, we had to stop because the boat could go no further. The sleek, long wooden boats – *chalanas* – drew up to the side of our boat; after some discussion, we started to unload our gear into the *chalanas*. These boats held sizable loads despite the appearance that they floated

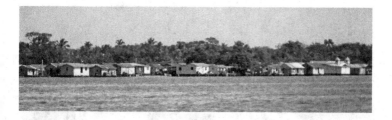

Figure 9.3 Arriving at stilt village in Lagunetas.

low in the water. Cameras, videos, notebooks, medical supplies, sleeping gear were all unloaded, and by the time everything was into the boats it was late afternoon.

Off we headed over the waves into a lagoon that appeared deserted until, in the distance, we could see houses on the water (Figure 9.3). As we approached the town of about 20 buildings, more people on boats came to greet us and accompany us the rest of the way. The houses were about three feet above the water, on stilts. Most were one-room structures with a large, uncovered porch. Walls and roofs were mostly corrugated tin. The size varied from 8 by 10 to 10 by 15 feet and might house 8–16 people. Some had small pens for pigs (Figure 9.4). At night, the family slept in layers of hammocks crisscrossing the room. The biggest building was actually a small store with a generator and a large wraparound porch with a bench. Adults and children thronged to the porch to see what we were about. They greeted us warmly and brought us dinner of fish and potatoes. To them, we were tall, pale, somewhat clumsy people who didn't speak much Spanish and had trouble balancing on their boats. They were shorter than us and their skin darkly tanned. Some had blonde hair and freckles. They were amazed at us foreigners and all the equipment we unloaded.

When we asked about the possibility of staying on the store porch for the night, they generously told us that they would do their best to accommodate us. They cheerfully gave us a boat tour

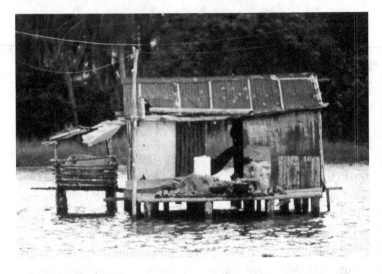

Figure 9.4 Typical house of corrugated steel walls and roof, wooden porch for cooking, nets and salt fish and a small enclosure for a pig.

of the town – Nancy in front, welcoming and hugging people. Most of the porches had mounds of salted fish prepared for sale and many held fires for cooking fish and stew. The inside of the typical house was a bare floor with a stove on one side and a tiny table. The 'toilet' was a small hole in the floor. Colorful metal dishes were arranged on racks on the walls. In a corner, washed, clean clothes hung on hangers. One family had a pet monkey and another kept cormorants as pets. Cormorants are long-necked birds that are excellent at fishing. The people put a string around its throat so it couldn't swallow the fish it had caught; the owner of the pet bird simply reached into its neck to take out the fish and then the bird dove down for another.

The next day, we roused ourselves – Steve slept in a mesh hammock and the rest of us were on the porch floor. We made ourselves some breakfast, and as we were eating, boats from the town carrying children and adults docked at the store and hung around the porch. Clearly, this was a special occasion: Men and women had bathed in the lake, washed their hair and brushed their teeth and then put on their nicest clothes. The women had also powdered themselves.

Nancy gathered people together and spoke about what the villagers called *El Mal* (the evil). She explained that it was an illness inherited from parent to child. She also explained that the sickness was worldwide, and *her* mother had it as well. That meant she and they were part of the same family and that she hoped they would agree to be part of a study to find the cause and hopefully treatment. She had given blood and skin samples too and showed them the scar on her arm from the skin biopsy. She patiently answered all the questions people had. This, of course, was new information for the family. They had thought that *El Mal* was unique to them. They believed that every child of a parent with HD had inherited the disease but that only some children actually showed symptoms. Nancy taught them rudimentary genetics so they could understand the inherited aspects of the disease. She was so persuasive that everyone agreed to help.

We set up an examining table against the outside wall of the store and hung a tarp as a backdrop so Steve could film while I did examinations. To the side, was a low table where we put papers and pedigree. A pedigree is simply a diagram of the family tree that geneticists construct when studying people with inherited diseases. Symbols are used to show relationships between family members and indicate which individuals have certain genetic pathogenic variants, traits and diseases within a family as well as vital status. We had to constantly update this family tree as we examined more and more people. Inside, we set up a place to draw blood and take skin biopsies of the people in town. We obtained written consent and a polaroid picture from each person.

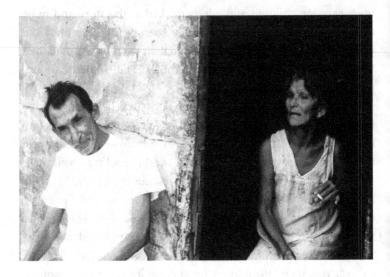

Figure 9.5 Venezuelan couple who both had HD and had 14 living children together.

Steve and I worked like clockwork, examining and filming everybody in the HD families, which included all the children of the so-called 'double dose' family as well as their cousins (Figure 9.5). Except for those that obviously were showing HD symptoms, I found only an eight-year-old cousin who looked like he had young onset HD. I felt I had really given each person in the town a thorough exam. I found no one of the 'double dose' family to have a new or more severe disease. A 'double' dose was either lethal, by chance didn't exist or was the same as a 'single' dose. Getting this data, I knew, was a very important part of the project.

The geneticists had emphasized that it was important to determine if HD is or is not a truly dominant disease. For another dominantly inherited disease, familial hypercholesterolemia (that gives people strokes and heart attacks in early adulthood), inheriting two copies of the mutant gene had been shown to cause strokes and heart attacks in children. This observation allowed the investigators to find the cause of the disease. Their work resulted in the Nobel Prize. Perhaps something similar would prove true in HD. But after our work that day, it appeared that either two HD genes did not lead to a new or more severe disease or none of the 14 children had two HD genes. I felt good about the job I had done – particularly since Steve and I had had such a problem before and I had almost ruined the first trip to this amazing town. Nancy and I never talked further about what would have happened to the project if the Lagunetas trip was canceled. For Nancy, it had all worked out in the end and everything else was water under the bridge and not worth dwelling on. Always forward.

We left Lagunetas in the late afternoon to return to Maracaibo on the Coast Guard boat. It was a five-hour trip. The usual fierce evening winds and the waves were against us. Waves crashed over the bow and against the sides of the boat. Everything was drenched and Steve had to find a dry place for his equipment as there was little that wasn't soaked by the time we got back. I was happy the trip went according to plan, but I hoped that in the future we could stay longer in Lagunetas and get to know the family better. I also realized that Nancy was as comfortable in remote places as she was in NIH boardrooms or at Julie Andrew's house. She was an unstoppable force. I was in awe of her but was frustrated that I hadn't had a chance to get to know her better.

Two days later, I left Venezuela having had one of the truly memorable times of my life. Jack was jealous when I told him how the trip had gone. He wanted to be part of any adventure that I had. Jack could see how thrilling the trip had been and said he hoped to be part of the Venezuelan project too.

10

. . . . .

Exploring
the Neurotransmitters
of Basal Ganglia

Despite the short trip to Venezuela, back in Michigan, I had to return to the lab work. It took several weeks to fully get back in the rhythm of things. The Venezuela experience was on the forefront of my mind. I had seen poverty in Appalachia and Chicago but the poverty in Venezuela was new to me and of a different magnitude. The abject lack of resources and support was depressing. I was motivated to continue with the project and work hard in our own lab to understand the cause of the illness. I also wanted to get to know Nancy better and work side by side with her in her efforts.

Jack and I continued working on the grant we had obtained when Ellen was born. Our aim was to identify the neurotransmitters of the motor pathways that influence the disorderly movements of Parkinson's and Huntington's disease. As is the case in many laboratory experiments, the current technology limited what we could and could not do. The discovery of the microscope had opened up avenues for understanding biology previously invisible to the naked eye. Similarly, lab work in basic science means keeping up with and understanding the latest in imaging technology. Then it's up to investigators to figure out the techniques for applying that technology. Often, it's the scientists themselves who innovate new techniques or even discover new technologies – necessity being the mother of invention.

In our case, Jack and I realized that doing the neurochemical work on the motor system not only was challenging but also demanded a lot of experimental animals – rats. Many of our experiments required us making a lesion in the brain, waiting for several weeks, then often making a second lesion in the brain, and finally killing the animal by rapid decapitation, removing the brain and making tiny little punches in the tissue to use for the final neurochemical measures. A mistake at any point wrecked the experiment. Furthermore, the amount of tissue we got from each animal was so small we often had to pool the tissues of several animals together for a sufficient measure. If we mixed animals with good lesions with those that weren't so good, then the whole experiment flopped. We didn't know whether the lesions were good until after the experiment was finished.

In order to get around these problems, we needed a better technique to answer our questions. We had already begun to work on measuring neurotransmitter receptors autoradiographically in sections of brain tissue. An autoradiograph is a photographic image, similar to an image on an x-ray film, that is produced by radiation and is often used with $[^{14}C]$ or $[^{125}I]$ to image the location of different brain functions. My old friends from Sol Snyder's lab, Candace Pert and Mike Kuhar, had devised a way of doing receptor autoradiography on very thin tissue sections. With their method, a thin tissue section was placed on a microscope slide and incubated with a radioactively labeled chemical. Some of the chemical bound to the neurotransmitter receptors on the tissue, and the excess, unbound chemical could be rinsed off. If a coverslip coated in a photographic emulsion was applied against the tissue section for a few weeks, and then developed, a picture appeared of the receptors on the brain section.

It was a neat method but it was not for us. We needed to have a method that was less complicated to execute and could actually measure the *number* of receptors. Receptor numbers change after lesioning the different pathways in the motor system. Anyone who has used the zoom function on a smartphone understands the notion of getting greater definition and detail. If we had more definition and detail and could measure the number of receptors, we could presumably then determine which pathways were most important in a circuit. This was crucial.

Jack and I had used the film autoradiography method to study brain sugar metabolism which involved [^{14}C]-radioactively labeled sugar (glucose). For these experiments, we didn't need emulsion-coated coverslips; we could use regular x-ray film. The images on the x-ray film had great definition and showed a lot of detail. We could see all the tiny regions of the brain that we were interested in. But we couldn't use regular x-ray film to measure the neurotransmitter receptors because the receptor studies used tritium [^{3}H] – a radioactive isotope of hydrogen that was too weak for normal x-ray film.

As we were trying to figure out the most efficient way to conduct our experiments, we learned that a company had recently released a new type of x-ray film that was sensitive to the weaker energy, tritium. This new type of film was not yet widely used and its applications therefore not known. We were early adopters; we decided to try working with the new film to see if it would give us the information we wanted. We dipped the tissue sections in [^{3}H]-labeled receptor drugs, rinsed them off and dried them quickly with a hairdryer. We applied them against the tritium-sensitive x-ray film, waited several weeks and developed the film in the darkroom.

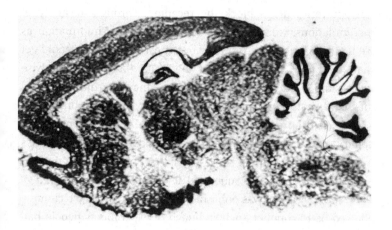

Figure 10.1 Autoradiogram of glutamate receptors in rat brain.

The darker the area of the image, the more receptors. The left side is the front of the brain and the right side the back with the cerebellum (the dark horn-like structure) and the brainstem below it. The dark areas are grains on a film; there is no tissue underneath.

It worked beautifully! Eureka! The greater definition allowed us to see all the anatomical details of the receptor distribution in the brain. This method was much easier, less prone to error, and most of all, more accurate than either of the previous methods (Figure 10.1). We used the method to look at all the GABA, glutamate, glycine, acetylcholine and dopamine receptors in rat, cat, monkey and human brains. If one damaged a group of nerve cells, we could see receptors locally and downstream changed as a result. We could quantitate the changes numerically and determine which pathways influenced others.

Next, we needed to figure out how to measure the number of receptors. We devised a type of radioactive yardstick (or standard) by mixing known amounts of radioactivity with brain tissue and applying these standards to the same piece of film as the slides of tissue sections. Using the radioactive standards, we could calculate the number of receptors in any given area. We could also see how powerful drugs block the receptor. Through a variety of manipulations, we not only got all the chemical information as we had previously in a test tube but, most importantly, could get that data from tiny regions of the brain that were otherwise impossible to study. We could do very fancy pharmacology and lots of other studies using these thin sections of frozen brain.

We used the new technique to measure GABA receptors. We could do all sorts of experiments you couldn't do with Candace's method. We wrote a first short paper describing the new method and its application and submitted it to the *European Journal of Pharmacology* and it was published on June 2, 1981. The technique allowed us to conduct a whole bunch of experiments people had never done before. This new approach quickly superseded the prior popular 'grind and bind technique' commonly used – grinding up tissue and throwing in the radioactivity to see how much binds. In a way, we were explorers like Lewis and Clarke. Everything was there, but it took us recording it to map it for everybody else. Scientists knew one part of the brain sent nerve endings to another, but they didn't know which pathways were most important or the chemicals used as neurotransmitters. When I began working in Sol's lab not much was known. In Michigan, we started studies to identify, define and map many of the neurotransmitters in the motor system.

We also wrote up a more detailed description of our new method and its application to the study of neurotransmitter receptors after specific brain lesions. We submitted the longer paper to *Science* and the editors sent it out for supposedly 'anonymous' peer reviews. One review was very positive, and the second review essentially said, what's the big deal? (Only big deals get published in *Science*.) So, it was rejected. We were dismayed; we thought our new method was certainly a big deal, both in and of itself and for the new experiments it opened up. Obviously we had other places than *Science* to publish and we did what any good academic does: We began readying the manuscript for submission elsewhere.

That's about when I got a call from Candace. "Hey, Anne! How are things? I saw your manuscript for *Science*." Her voice trailed off. "Miles got it for review."

Miles was Miles Herkenham, a scientist who Candace was working with at the National Institutes of Health. Miles, our reviewer who was no longer anonymous, had shared our paper with her. Candace sounded especially excited. "Neat method," she said. "We tried to make it work but couldn't until we got your manuscript and we read how you did it. Now we have it working. Did you see the latest *Nature*? No? That's *our* picture on the cover using *your* method! It's really cool!"

Before I could catch my breath she delivered her final zinger. "I'm sorry Miles was so negative in his review but I'm sure you can get the paper published somewhere else. How is everything going with you otherwise?"

I ended the call as soon as I could. I was in shock. I could understand ignoring the whole anonymous reviewer business but how did she have the nerve to basically steal a method that was original to Jack and me? I considered her a friend. She and Miles were considered reputable scientists. Ironically, Candace had let everyone know how unfair she thought it was that Sol Snyder, as head of the Hopkins Lab and according to established norms, was the one who received the Lasker prize for the discovery of the opiate receptor when she believed she was the one responsible.

I picked up the phone again, called the editor at *Science* and told him the whole story. "Take a look at the cover of the new *Nature*," I said. He said he had a copy on his desk but hadn't looked at it yet. I waited while he shuffled some papers around. He coughed. "I get it," he said. "Consider your paper accepted with us."

It wasn't as bad as it could've been. Jack and I had published something on our method in the *European Journal of Pharmacology*. The method that Jack and I described became widely used by the rest of the scientific community so eventually all the silliness became irrelevant but to this day I have trouble understanding why Candace did what she did. Competition and academic rivalries are part of the game but undercutting one's allies has always seemed counterproductive as well as unethical.

Those first several years, Jack and I worked nonstop. For our own mental health and for some family time, we needed breaks from time to time to get away. Fortunately, during Christmas and the girls' spring breaks from school we were able to vacation in the Bahamas. In the late 1970s, my parents and my brother had bought a share of a large piece of property in the Bahamas – about a quarter of a small island off Eleuthera – Harbour Island. It had a beautiful, old Bahamian home at the crest of land between the harbor side and the ocean side of the island. It had land opening onto a five-mile pink, coral sand beach. As a relative of a member of the club of shareholders, I could rent one or two rooms in the house or the 'dock house.' It was a great place for a vacation. Every night, a wonderful Bahamian dinner would be on the table. A little sunburn to top it off and you could have a wonderful tropical evening.

Then in the early 1980s, my family bought a home with another family in the club. It had an attic where we kept our windsurfer. My dad had a small motorboat and a 26-foot sloop. The place was heaven. The girls loved it and so did Jack. He got buckets and shovels and put on the sunscreen and went off with them to the beach. He dug in the sand with them and taught them how to ride the waves.

My father rigged a fish tank that circulated seawater. It sat on the edge of a gazebo that was built down by the bay. From there you could walk out in the tidal shallows and catch small fish, shrimp and crabs. Once Jack and I and the girls were fishing in tidal pools on the oceanside when suddenly something moved. I slapped my net over it. It was a small octopus! It was a real rascal and had to be held down in the bucket with a top. We made it

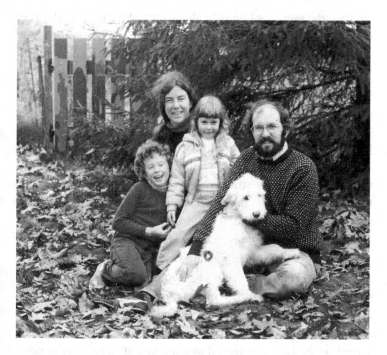

Figure 10.2 Jessie, me, Ellen, Molly (the dog) and Jack about 1983 in our yard in Michigan. The garden gate the girls painted is in the background.

back to the aquarium and put him in. The fish freaked. They hid in any crevice they could find. The next day we found out why. Little skeletons floated around in the tank and the octopus seemed very satisfied.

The girls were growing up (Figure 10.2). I didn't want them to see themselves as victims and I wanted them to have the smarts to stick up for themselves if problems arose at school. When Ellen came home one day complaining that one of the boys in her class snuck into her desk every day and snitched her bag of popcorn, I told her to tell him off but Ellen said she was afraid he'd hit her. My father would have told her what he told me – how to make a fist and punch the boy between the eyes, but I thought about what else she could do. The popcorn was more than an optional treat for Ellen. She was a night person who woke up late and just didn't feel like eating much breakfast in the morning so Joan had her take a snack to school every day to keep her from getting too hungry before lunchtime.

"Why don't you sprinkle your popcorn with cayenne pepper and wait and see what happens," I suggested. At first Ellen protested and was alarmed at this aggressive tactic but I assured her that after all it was *her* popcorn, and nobody should be messing with it. She tried my strategy and was jubilant when she came home from school! Her popcorn had indeed been snitched and she saw the culprit distressed at the drinking fountain later that day. Problem solved: Her popcorn wasn't taken again.

Maybe because of how well the cayenne popcorn incident had turned out, Ellen began to develop her own entrepreneurial strategies when it seemed necessary to solve a problem. One evening when Ellen was in second grade, Jessie was complaining at the dinner table because as a fourth grader and member of the school band, she was required to sell a box of candy bars to raise money for the band. Since our house wasn't really in a neighborhood and few houses were around, she didn't see how she could sell them. Ellen asked how much they cost. Jessie said she had 40 and had to sell them for 50 cents apiece.

Ellen thought briefly and then said, "I'll buy them."

We all looked at her. I thought, "Is she nuts?"

After dinner, Ellen went downstairs and came out of her room with $20 in small bills she had saved over the last year. She gave it to Jessie and took the candy. Both Jack and I were stunned but Ellen said she wasn't worried about selling them.

The next evening, Ellen said she had sold half the candy already and was going to make a profit. She'd taken 20 candy bars to school with her and waited until the bus ride home to sell them for a dollar a piece.

The next day, she sold the rest and the only mistake she made was that she sold two on a loan and was never paid back. She learned about the risks associated with loans but everything worked out fine: The band got their $20 contribution, Jessie was happy to get the dreaded chore off her back and Ellen made a handsome profit. From then on, I have relentlessly teased Ellen about her natural talent for business and ruthless capitalism.

All the while, Jack and I discussed at home or on long walks how we thought the brain controlled movement. Anatomists and physiologists had written about pathways connecting regions of the brain but how they functioned was still a mystery. We knew that people with Parkinson's disease had a dopamine loss in the striatum due to death of dopamine nerve cells in the 'black substance' (substantia nigra) of the brainstem that sends dopamine input to the striatum. I could never forget that time in medical school when I had personally witnessed how a tiny pill – that served as a dopamine replacement in the brain of a person with Parkinson's disease – could lead to such dramatic improvement in Parkinson's symptoms. Was there a missing neurotransmitter in Huntington's diseased brain? The section of the basal ganglia known as the striatum was known to be damaged in Huntington's. Three scientific groups, including Patrick and Edith McGeer, who were a couple who collaborated on experiments like Jack and I did, published articles within months of each other reporting that the enzyme synthesizing GABA was very decreased in Huntington's striatum. Could 'GABA replacement' restore normal function to patients suffering from Huntington's (Figure 10.3)?

Ira Shoulson, who Jack and I knew because of his work on HD, set up a first-class definitive study to answer this question. He was a couple years older than us and had trained in neurology at the University of Rochester and then spent two years at the National Institutes of Health training in experimental therapeutics and clinical trial design. We admired what he was doing and Jack

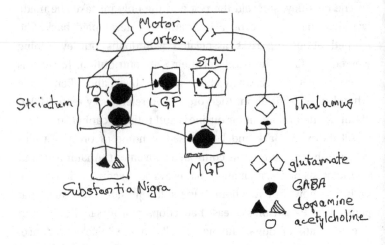

Figure 10.3 Schematic of motor circuit we helped define.

Abbreviations: LGP – lateral globus pallidus; MGP – medial globus pallidus; STN – subthalamic nucleus. Black objects with small dark endings at the ends of their processes are inhibitory onto the nerve cells they connect with. The open objects are excitatory onto cells they contact.

went out of his way to work with him; they soon became fast friends. Ira and a colleague published a clinical severity scale for Huntington's disease that evaluated a person's capacity to work, live independently and take care of oneself or the need for someone else's care. The scale was simple and could be used to follow the progression of a patient's illness.

Unlike dopamine, there was no medication to directly increase brain GABA but there were drugs that could mimic GABA at the GABA receptors. Ira was studying whether the GABA-enhancing drug baclofen could improve HD symptoms and actually slow the progression of the disease. However, Ira's study showed that replacing GABA function did *not* improve HD symptoms. Why was that?

At the time, the striatal nerve cells were known to use GABA as a neurotransmitter. The GABA cells sent processes to synapse with another group of neurons. But what about the transmitter of *the other group of nerve cells contacted* by the GABA striatal cells? At the time, it was unknown.

Jack and I decided we could perform an experiment to determine the neurotransmitter of the next nerve cells in the pathway. Jack made tiny lesions deep in the rats' brain to wipe out the cells that received input from the striatum. My job was then to determine which potential neurotransmitter was missing.

The study turned out to be quick and easy. The neurotransmitter was also GABA.

Now it all made sense. GABA is inhibitory – suppressing the action of the cell it contacts. In other words, the striatal GABA cells inhibit the next cells, which are also using GABA to connect with the cells they contact. A double negative. That was why Ira's study had found that replacing the GABA didn't have any impact. GABA replacement boosted *both* pathways – thereby canceling each other out. Eliminating a possibility, especially one that seemed obvious, and then finding out why it wouldn't work was another big deal of a breakthrough.

We took stock of how far we'd come and where we needed to go next. Our experiments in the lab had now identified the neurotransmitters of two important pathways – the corticospinal tract (glutamate) and the pallidothalamic pathway (GABA). The next big question we needed to answer: How did these pathways play a role in movement?

In our discussions of patients and how they moved, Jack and I realized that although contemporary textbooks and academic articles described Parkinson's patients as slow and unable to move, that was not how we saw our patients. We observed that rather than moving slowly, they had difficulty with 'switching' behaviors. Once sitting, they were slow to stand up. Once walking, they had trouble stopping. Tapping fingers was slow at first but then got faster and faster. Parkinson's was not so much a disease of slowness, we hypothesized, but rather a positive feedback loop in the brain that reinforced ongoing behavior and made it hard to switch to a new behavior. Perhaps dopamine, which was diminished in Parkinson's, was necessary for switching behaviors not for speed.

Huntington's disease was different. When patients performed a particular task or behavior, such as moving an arm or a leg, unwanted movements interrupted the ongoing task. Maintaining a behavior was difficult because other behaviors randomly intervened.

Ultimately, in both diseases fine motor coordination was impaired.

How did these different diseases affect the brain's pathways? We began to put together diagrams of the pathways or circuits that were thought to play a role. The neurotransmitters of only some of the pathways were known. We began to investigate the unknown pathways by lesioning first one pathway or another and then observing what happened chemically to neurotransmitter levels and receptors. All these studies were done in rats but thanks to the generosity of our patients and their families we also had a human brain bank. Jack became an expert at taking whole sections of the human brain for autoradiography (Figure 10.4). Things that we learned from animal studies could be checked in human brains.

Students and fellows in our lab led different experiments, and each brought their own perspective. Helen Pan (my first graduate student) led experiments on GABA receptors, Tim Greenamyre (my first MD/PhD student) worked on glutamate receptors and Roger Albin (a postdoctoral fellow) on pathways in Huntington's disease. The lab was always hopping, students worked all night with the music playing.

Unlike Jack who was quiet and mild-mannered, I was often getting myself in trouble for my aggressive behavior. Something would come over me; I was like a pot boiling over. The second year I was a faculty member at the University of Michigan, I had

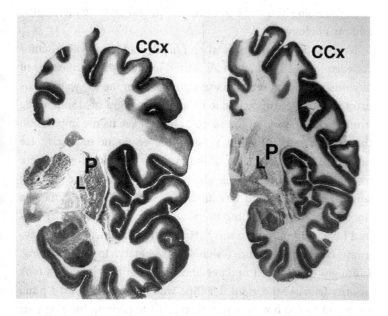

Figure 10.4 Autoradiograms of GABA receptors in whole hemisphere sections of a normal control brain (left) and HD brain (right).

The receptors are generally normal in both except the area marked P for putamen, a key area of the striatum that degenerates in HD. The decreased intensity in this area of HD brain indicates a loss of nerve cells and their receptors. Of interest is the increased intensity of the area marked L (the lateral globus pallidus) compared to the L area of the normal brain. The increased density indicates an increase in receptors on pallidal neurons because of the loss of GABA input from the putamen. The cerebral cortex (CCx) is the surface of the brain and is fairly normal.

a blowup with a faculty member of the physical medicine and rehabilitation department. I had asked for a specific study to be carried out and the faculty member had completely ignored it.

That evening, when he came up to the ward to talk to me, I made sure I verbally abused him in front of medical students and nurses. The words seemed to spontaneously jump out of my mouth. I was again the kid; I got carried away. Understandably, this doctor went back to the chair of his department and complained that I had been harassing him. Sid had to call me in and mediate the dispute and my apology.

My next big blowout was when I finally had it out with a senior colleague named George. It all started because of a confluence of circumstances. George's lab was right next to mine. He watched us extra carefully. He appeared to be afraid we might steal something from his laboratory. At the same time, he gave us the impression that he felt vastly superior to us in the academic hierarchy. He never seemed to lose sight of the fact that Jack and I were mere assistant professors and he was a full professor. He called my senior technician, who was 30 years old, 'boy'. Then came the final straw. I was finishing the touches on a big grant that Jack and I were submitting to the NIH and the deadline was two days away. George, Jack and I shared a secretary. In the morning, I brought her the text updates and I told her that this work took priority because the grant deadline was so close. Around 1 p.m., I went in to see how she was doing and to pick up the first part of the text so I could briefly go over it. She hadn't worked on the grant at all! She said that just after I had come in, George had come in and demanded that she enter this week's references into his database. She said she was afraid not to comply. I immediately sought out George and got into an aggressive argument with him.

Sid called the next day to ask me to meet in his office with George. Oh, man! Not again. I had to apologize to George and agree not to threaten him again.

My schedule included seeing two half days of patients a week. One half day was for supervising residents and fellows who were seeing movement disorder patient cases. The other half day I saw my private patients. Both Jack and I communicated closely with our patients – often spontaneously calling them up on the phone to check on their well-being. Patients or their families occasionally wrote to us requesting a second opinion. Sometimes patients wrote to us out of the blue. Often, these letters described things they found particularly frustrating. Sometimes, patients wrote direct criticisms of us as doctors and at other times they praised our attention and care. We tried to do the job as best we knew how and learned to take it all – the criticism and praise – in stride.

In keeping with this, I received a thick letter one day. It was handwritten on both sides of eight sheets of paper. The handwriting was neat but somewhat shaky, suggesting that the writer was older. She introduced herself as the mother of a patient who was booked to see me in one month. She wanted to summarize her daughter's case for me.

The daughter was a family physician who had what we then called severe manic-depressive disorder (now called bipolar disorder) and according to her mother had had numerous flare-ups of her illness over the past 20 years. I began to dread seeing this patient – particularly because her mother would probably come to the appointment which would be long and complicated. So, when the day came, I was in a bad mood. At the assigned time, I went to get the patient from the waiting room and a pleasant-looking woman stood up – alone – no mother. She had come in from Ypsilanti State Hospital accompanied by two security people. Ypsilanti State is the Michigan facility for the criminally insane and for others who have no means but need long-term care on a locked ward.

The woman was very articulate and quickly told me she had noted some uncontrollable movements of her lips and tongue. She knew that these could be side effects of her medication and wanted my opinion on which medications were the least harmful for her long term. She was very pleasant and precise. We finished in only 20 minutes, and I had 40 minutes left on my schedule.

"So . . . why are you in Ypsilanti State?" I asked naively.

It was as if I had plugged her into an electric socket. The woman became incredibly animated and said she was so glad to know that 'we' were on her side. She praised us for having the *Time* magazine in the waiting room that reported all the excitement in the astrology world over the upcoming harmonic convergence of evangelicals. This event, she told me, indicated that the prophets were coming to an extraordinary end. Her excitement was contagious, and I began to feel thrilled myself.

Then she went into her history – how she'd landed at Ypsilanti State Hospital. She said she had been living on an upper floor of Huron Towers – the only high-rise in Ann Arbor – and doing well when she began to get signals from a guy in Kansas and other signals from another guy in the Middle East about collaborating to bring Jesus, Muhammed and Buddha together in nearby Detroit. She said she had what she called 'upper shockers' (imaginary metal antennae on her head capable of delivering extreme electrical power) and planned with two others to focus electrical power to destroy Jesus, Muhammad and Buddha all at once. She said she had equipment in her apartment that altered the electric and magnetic fields around the top of Huron Towers and it became so powerful that the police decided to investigate. The police arrested her after having found her enormous generators and other equipment. But she had not given up hope. She was still trying to use her upper shockers to get the three religious prophets together to change the world. She apologized that she and her collaborators had to damage large sections of Detroit in order to accomplish her goals, but it just had to be! She went on and on about her plans.

I finished her appointment on time, and she went back to Ypsilanti on new medication, but she left a big impression on me. I realized that *I* now wanted upper shockers. It was infectious. She had transferred her excitement to me. Since this encounter, I have often wished I could grow my own upper shockers. I imagined them looking like those metal antennae stuck to headbands that kids wear at Halloween. What a cool concept – to have two upper shockers on the top of your head that can pivot, focus and put out powerful shock waves to eliminate your enemies. I realized how amazing the human mind is and how it can be supercharged, however stressful that may be. I also realized how often I had felt supercharged. Years later, diagnosed as bipolar, I was able to label that supercharged feeling as hypomania. My diagnosis would also explain my bouts of aggressive behavior and hopeless depression. Thank goodness I was finally treated.

Of course, the human mind can become charged in ways that are truly sad. My patients with Huntington's went through such hell with their disease that suicide was not a completely irrational notion. In fact, the suicide rate in Huntington's disease is about 7 percent, well above the national average. I was not very astute psychiatrically but over time I got better at talking about depression and suicide each time a patient came to see me. One patient was an elegant woman in the first stage of the illness. Her major problem was auditory hallucinations that plagued her constantly. Interestingly, the hallucinations were not voices telling her to kill herself but rather loud and unbearable music. She couldn't stand it. Nothing stopped them. She got more and more depressed. I tried to help by prescribing antidepressants, neuroleptics and anticonvulsants, but none of them worked. She told me she was going to kill herself. She had stashed away pills and she planned to take them. I called a friend in psychiatry and we had her admitted to the psychiatric ward. There, nothing seemed to work either. The doctors gave her electroshock treatments. They didn't work.

This woman had a sister who came to visit her frequently in the hospital. This sister was two years older than my patient and hadn't seen a doctor about Huntington's disease, but when I bumped into her in the hospital, I could tell immediately from her choreic (dance-like) movements that she was definitely affected by the disease as well. My patient's husband, her sister and her sister's husband were all very attentive and I spent hours talking to all four of them about how things would get better. My patient was not badly affected from the motor standpoint, and so if the hallucinations and depression could be managed, her quality of life would improve. There are no cures for HD but aspects of the illness – depression, chorea, irritability and hallucinations – can be helped by medication.

But the patient wanted to be released from the hospital although she was still quite sick. She wanted a ruling from a judge about whether or not she could be released. Both the psychiatrist and I wanted her to stay longer until her mental health had improved, but the judge ruled that she was free to go. Her sister picked her up from the hospital.

The next day, the husband called to tell me that his wife and her sister had disappeared. As far as the two husbands could figure out, they had packed up small suitcases and disappeared in one of their cars. The police were put on the case. Their car was found at the Detroit airport and a ticket agent was found who said the two women had asked her where a nice quiet place was to spend a few days. She'd recommended Fort Wayne, Indiana. Three days later, after a really hot weekend, the husband called to tell me that both women had been found. Dead in a hotel room.

Oh, God.

The medical examiner called and told me that since they were suicides, they would have a full autopsy but that the husbands had asked if the brains could be donated for research. I, of course, said that they would be very valuable and that we had a brain bank that would make sure the tissues were used for a good cause. The autopsy found high levels of antidepressants and barbiturates in each of them. The brains were frozen as soon as possible after the autopsy but there was already some decomposition since they had lain locked in their hotel room for two days. As it turned out, the brains proved very valuable and showed for the first time what receptor changes in early HD looked like and how these changes could generate a new hypothesis of what goes wrong in HD.

This event threw me into a deep depression. I felt responsible for the deaths. I felt sick. How could I have allowed her to go home? Especially with her sister who was also quite depressed. If only I had gone directly before the judge myself and explained the situation maybe I could have saved them. If only I had been able to get the hallucinations under control earlier the whole thing wouldn't have happened. Had I recognized her depression soon enough, her mental pain could have been nipped in the bud. I should have insisted she see a psychiatrist instead of acting like I could take care of it myself. Shit. I had killed two women. I shouldn't be a doctor. I should be dead. I woke up every night about 2 a.m. and couldn't stop worrying about all the things I should have done or said or been. I'd fall asleep again about 4 a.m. and wake up two hours later, tired and consumed by a profound sense of worthlessness. Anything could make me cry. I wanted to die. I lost weight. I cursed the kids and Jack. I went to bed early only to wake up anxious and panicked. I drank too much. I woke up with visions of double-sided blades going through my heart and blood spurting out all over. I started checking the blades of the knives in the house. It was early summer, but everything was bleak, colorless, smell-less, tasteless. Nothing was worth loving – most of all me.

The worst thing was the kids. They seemed to think they had done something wrong. Jack knew what I had gone through, and he knew how depressed I was. He'd wrap himself around me in bed in the morning and tell me that it wasn't my fault, that I wasn't responsible for their deaths and that the women would have found a way no matter what. He reminded me of the higher suicide rates among Huntington's patients, but it didn't help. I couldn't believe him. I'd often push him away and refuse to make love. I let him see me cry, but I didn't let him know that I wanted to stick a knife into my body. He encouraged me to see someone, but I didn't want to. After my college experience, I didn't trust psychiatrists. Jack didn't push it because he had seen me even more depressed before and he knew it eventually passed. I wanted to die and believed I was worthless, but from past experiences, including the time in college, I also recognized that I was depressed and knew that even if it lasted months, the depression would go away. By then Nancy had become close to me and the rest of the family and helped me to handle things with the kids. They were so young – three and five. She told me to tell them directly how depressed I was and why and that it was nothing they had done. I told them I loved them, and I would start feeling better soon.

The kids responded by taking care of *me* – setting the table, being good about helping to get dressed and ready for school in the morning. Slowly, I improved and could get pleasure from things around me. However, my self-image was always low, and more often than not I thought I should be dead. Later, I was treated for my mood disorder.

11

• • • • •

Functional Anatomy of Basal Ganglia Disorders

The work in our lab progressed as we tried to understand the pathways in the brain that led to the disorderly movements we saw in our patients suffering with Huntington's and Parkinson's diseases. As we worked through the neural circuits, we lesioned one area in the rat brain and then measured the receptors affected by the removal of the pathway. Helen Pan worked by making lesions of the dopamine pathway, the pathway affected in Parkinson's disease. We predicted that dopamine lesions would remove inhibition of the nerve cells in the striatum making them more excitable. Helen found, however, that dopamine appeared to be *inhibiting* or *decreasing* the firing of some nerve cells but *exciting* or *increasing* firing in the others. How can this be? How could one transmitter have opposite effects on the striatal nerve cells? Our original hypothesis of how the pathways connected and affected each other didn't take this differential effect into account.

Jack and I had read articles on the effects of dopamine on striatal cells written by scientists recording electrical activity in the striatum. They said that dopamine was excitatory, not inhibitory. An important group of investigators studying this problem was at Michigan State University – just an hour's drive from Ann Arbor. Highly regarded basal ganglia electrophysiologists Steve Kitai and Charlie Wilson spent an afternoon with us showing their data. Dopamine definitely seemed to be exciting some striatal nerve cells when an electrode in the cell recorded the reaction to applied dopamine. As a pharmacologist, however, I knew that dopamine inhibited some other cells as well. There now appeared to be at least two kinds of dopamine receptors – D1 excitatory receptors and D2 inhibitory receptors.

As we pondered these problems, other investigators were studying two peptides (short proteins) that could function as neurotransmitters in the striatum. One peptide was called enkephalin (one of our brain's own opiates – discovered in part by Candace Pert and Sol Snyder). Enkephalin was highly concentrated in the striatal nerve cells that also contain GABA. These enkephalin/GABA cells connected to the neurons in the external part of the section of the brain called globus pallidus – a key link in the motor circuits. The other peptide, substance P, was also in striatal GABA cells but these cells projected back to the substantia nigra pars reticulata – another but different link in the anatomical circuit. Each peptide was present in about 50 percent of striatal neurons. All these neurons contained GABA. Enkephalin-containing neurons fed into different brain areas than substance P-containing neurons. Data also suggested that dopamine inhibits enkephalin cells through D2 dopamine receptors and excites substance P cells through D1 dopamine receptors.

While Helen was working on GABA receptors, Roger Albin began examining enkephalin and substance P pathways in the human HD brain in collaboration with Anton Reiner in the Michigan Anatomy

Department. Roger had been a neurology resident at Michigan and wanted to specialize in movement disorders. With his bushy beard and absent-minded professor approach to life, he was both brilliant and encyclopedic in his knowledge. He was more interested in the comparative anatomy of brain than Jack was. He obtained brains from turtles, snakes, cows and pigs. He studied these species just out of curiosity. Roger was always able to discuss obscure but relevant information. He teamed up with Anton Reiner who taught him the best method to stain enkephalin and substance P peptides with antibodies. The results imaged the peptide pathways. The two studied the peptides in human postmortem brains we had in our bank. With considerable effort examining many normal control and HD brains, Roger discovered that the enkephalin-containing striatal cells died first in Huntington's disease followed later by the substance P-containing neurons.

What appeared to happen under normal circumstances was that two interacting but separate pathways were coursing through the striatum. The two pathways controlled different aspects of movement. One pathway defined a positive feedback loop to reinforce ongoing behaviors and suppress unwanted movements. The other was important for fine motor coordination and for switching to new movements or activities.

On one of our trips to visit Jack's family in Boston, we decided to meet with Ann Graybiel, a professor at MIT, who was world-renowned for her descriptions of subpopulations of cells in the striatum that could be distinguished using different tissue stains. We found her to be brilliant, talkative and eager to discuss with us how she thought the basal ganglia might work. We shared with her our images of GABA, dopamine and other neurotransmitters in Huntington's brain. Our experiments complemented hers and we continued to discuss our respective findings and hypotheses with her over the course of our careers.

We were invited to give talks on our data at a symposium on basal ganglia research in Manchester, UK in 1986. There were scientists from all over the world presenting their work – including neurophysiological studies in Parkinsonian monkeys. These researchers were still trying to understand how their data made sense. They weren't thinking of the neurotransmitter actions but rather the electrical activity. Why did the electrical activity go up in some areas and down in others? How did the anatomy jibe with their results? Jack and I, however, could see a logical solution to their data based on what our data in rats and humans had taught us about the neurotransmitters of these pathways. The logical solution was that normally dopamine *decreased* the activity of enkephalin/GABA cells and *increased* the activity of substance P/GABA cells. The *loss* of dopamine resulted in the opposite: *increased* activity in enkephalin/ GABA cells and *decreased* activity in substance P/GABA cells. We discussed our thoughts with the other investigators and wrote up a summary of our hypothesis for the book produced by the symposium. Jack and I also wrote up our hypothesis for the first issue of the new journal *Movement Disorders* in 1986.

Back in the lab, Jack, Roger Albin and I began to work on specific experiments essentially challenging our model. After all, that was the whole point of a model. Could we find more data to support or reject it? As we collected more animal and human postmortem brain results, we modified and refined our model, adding and removing connections. Other investigators coined the terms 'direct' and 'indirect' pathways for the two circuits we had suggested. These two circuits were affected differently in Huntington's and Parkinson's diseases, and we used our hypothesis to suggest a cause of the different symptoms in the diseases. We collected evidence that the subthalamic nucleus, a tiny nucleus deep in the brain, was excitatory and used glutamate as a neurotransmitter. The subthalamic nucleus is a key component of the indirect pathway.

We had now identified the neurotransmitters of each pathway in the two circuits. Things were coming together.

In August 1987, the Michigan Chapter of the Committee to Combat Huntington's Disease hosted the annual meeting of the national organization in Ann Arbor. They asked Jack and I to participate and give talks to the attendees – who were mostly family members. About 200 people were scheduled to attend. Nancy was also going to be at the meeting, and we asked her to stay at our house.

The meeting was excellent.

The meeting ended on Sunday and Nancy came back to our house and played with the kids for a while before we took her to the airport in the late afternoon. Both Jessie and Ellen loved Nancy; she was fun to be with and was always interested in what they had to say. Jack and I sat outside in the yard drinking gin and tonics. It was a clear and beautiful day, warm in the high eighties. Then we all got into the car and headed to the airport. Jack was driving, I was a little giddy from the gin and tonic, and Nancy and the girls were in the back seat.

As we neared the airport, a huge ball of fire suddenly exploded before us! It was so large that it obliterated half the sky. It appeared to race from right to left across the road straight ahead of us. I had no idea where the explosion came from and Jack said, "Oh my god. That was a plane." The girls froze in horror as the ball of flames swept across the road about 300 feet in front of us and Jessie asked, "Are you sure?" Jack was certain. "It's the only thing it could be," he said. "And with that much fuel, it must have crashed on takeoff." Nancy gripped the girls' hands in the back seat. Seeing the magnitude of the conflagration, it seemed doubtful that anyone in the plane survived.

We could still take the exit to the airport because the explosion was just beyond it. We wanted to get off the road as soon as possible. We drove up to the Northwest Terminal and Nancy and I went inside while Jack and the girls waited in the car. People moved as usual through the check-in area, but as Nancy and I approached the counter, airport personnel could be seen in shock, crying. The atmosphere was eerie. We had seen the crash on the road but no one inside the terminal had seen it. The employees knew about it since they had been told over the phone. Remarkably the Northwest agent, teary-eyed, said she thought Nancy's flight would merely be delayed. The agents couldn't talk with us about the accident. I begged Nancy not to go. I didn't know what to say to the girls and she always knew what to do and what to say. Plus, I was fearful for her safety. Finally, I was able to persuade her to come back with us and leave the next day. When we got back to the car, the girls were so relieved that she was staying.

When we got back home, we turned on the TV. The accident was on every channel. Northwest Flight 255 to Phoenix had crashed on takeoff. So far there were no survivors. The TV showed gruesome pictures of the wreckage. We watched just long enough to learn what happened. Nancy stayed close to the girls, listening to their reactions and fear. She was remarkable. She didn't in any way try to minimize their emotions or the tragedy but rather talked to them openly and frankly and gently about what had happened. They listened intently, and I could see that she was able to calm them. Jack and I read each one a story and put them to bed.

Nancy was in the living room and she put the TV back on when Jack and I joined her. Everyone had died with the exception of a little girl whose mother died shielding her from the flames. The crash later turned out to be due to the pilot's failure to put the flaps down on takeoff. We were all afraid that someone from the Huntington's disease meeting was on the plane. The next morning, Nancy left to go back to New York. I called up the head of the chapter sponsoring the meeting, and he said that he knew of nobody from the meeting on the plane although they were still awaiting more information. As it turned out, there was no one. Jessie and Ellen emptied their piggy bank to send money to a relief fund for the lone surviving girl, and they were apprehensive the next time they took a flight. Thanks to Nancy, much of their trauma was relieved, but Jessie still avoids planes to this day.

I had to get over my own fears of flying as my career progressed, since I was often invited to speak on our work at other institutions. I was more gregarious and, at first, a better speaker than Jack, and so I often went to meetings alone and Jack stayed at home with the girls. One time, when I was in London giving a talk on glutamate in Alzheimer's disease at a symposium at the Royal Society, I called home at about 8 p.m. Ann Arbor time and Joan answered the phone.

"Is Jack there, Joan?"

"Uh . . . No, he's still in the hospital."

"He is? What's the problem? Is one of his patients sick?"

"Well . . . Uh . . . I don't know . . . I actually think he is in the emergency room."

"Really? What's he doing there?"

"Well . . . I think he's actually a patient in the emergency room." She sounded strangely calm, as if Jack had just gone out on an errand.

"What? What's wrong with him?" Obviously, I was alarmed. I'd just spoken to him the night before and he was fine.

"Well . . . Uh . . . he wasn't feeling great this morning and so he went to get checked out and called and said they were sending him to the ICU."

"What? The ICU? You're kidding! The ICU? That stands for Intensive Care Unit! Joan! I'm hanging up and calling the emergency room. I'll call you back later."

I hung up the phone and called the University of Michigan Hospital emergency room.

"This is Dr. Anne Young calling from London. Is Dr. John Penney a patient in the ER?"

"Uh . . . let me see . . . Why yes . . . yes, he's here."

"I want to speak to him or the doctor who's seeing him right away."

"Well . . . I think he's on his way to the ICU so maybe you should call there later."

"I'm his wife! I need to know what's wrong! Is he okay? What the hell is he doing there?" I was completely freaked out. I needed information.

"Now calm down. I'll see if I can find someone to talk to you."

"I'm calling from London. That's London, *England*!"

"Just a second. Hold on." There was a long pause.

"Dr. Young. Hi. I'm taking care of your husband. He's had a GI bleed and we're sending him to the ICU. He's stable and I can see if you can talk to him. Just a minute."

"Wait! Wait! A GI bleed? What's his crit?" A 'crit' is short for hematocrit – a measure of the amount of blood in your system. A normal level was 40.

"Well. It was 27 when he came in and he had no palpable blood pressure but now that he's hydrated up, his BP's okay and his crit is 20. He'll be getting blood transfusions in the ICU."

"Holy cow! Let me talk to him. Please." Another long pause, then fumbling with the phone.

"Hello?" I knew Jack's voice immediately. He sounded a bit odd and nasal.

"Jack? What's going on? Are you okay?"

"Well, I wasn't feeling great last night, and I got up in the middle of the night to take a shit but the bathroom was dark and I was all weak and sweaty. I didn't look at the shit and just went back to bed. This morning, I still felt really bad but I had clinic. I saw patients all morning and by noon I was really feeling bad, but I didn't have a fever or anything, so I did the afternoon teaching clinic. By the time I was done at 5 p.m., one of the residents said I looked terrible, and I really felt bad. I took another shit and saw that it was pitch black. I knew immediately that I had had a bleed.

200

I went to the ER and they did my crit and it was 27. They put in an IV and a big NG [nasogastric] tube and have been lavaging me with cold water down the tube. The blood is clearing and they're taking me to the ICU where they'll transfuse me. I'll be okay. I don't feel that bad."

"Jack. Does anyone know? It's 2 a.m. here and I'm coming home on a flight in the morning. I'm calling Roger and I'll call again before I leave. Jesus! Hang in there. I'll be there soon. I love you."

I hung up the phone and called Roger and told him to check up on Jack to make sure no one at the hospital was screwing up. From my experiences as a patient and as a doctor, I knew how easy it was for a tired, careless, forgetful or inexperienced health care worker to not understand what to do. Jack was stable when I called before my flight. When I got home, I went immediately to the hospital. I was relieved to learn that Jack had already been transferred from the ICU out to the floor. They had transfused him overnight and the bleeding had stopped. Looking at his stomach through an endoscope had shown lots of micro ulcers and inflammation.

That's when it came out that Jack had been suffering from migraines and instead of using more sensible therapy such as propranolol or ergots, he had treated his migraines with aspirin. About eight a day! He fessed up that recently he had developed what he had thought was a pulled muscle in his left back and so he was taking even more aspirin. About 12 a day! That 'pulled muscle' was, in fact, pain from the aspirin-induced stomach ulcers and he was making it worse by taking even more aspirin. For a long time after that he had to stop drinking coffee and alcohol and stay off chocolate. It was also the middle of the AIDS epidemic and a blood test to detect who was HIV positive had just been released a few months earlier, in March 1985. Blood transfusions were screened for HIV after that date but the recommendation for blood recipients was to be tested just after the transfusions and then again in six months to make sure undetectable degrees of infection had not been transmitted and reproduced. During those six months Jack and I had only protected sex. In those days, HIV was always fatal and although it was unlikely his transfusions were infected, there was every reason to be careful.

The lesson to the story, however, was that Jack had set the gold standard for clinic attendance at Michigan. When word got out about Jack's stoicism, Sid Gilman, the chair of neurology, expected everyone to see all their patients and perform all assigned teaching unless their hematocrit was less than 27.

In the midst of all this chaos at home, I learned from high school friends that Les Moore had been apprehended after seven years on the lam with the child. Les had abducted the child because she believed she was rescuing the child from an abusive situation. When the law caught up to her, the child was sent back to his biological mother. Les went to live at H.O.M.E. (Homeworkers Organized for More Employment), Inc. in Orland, Maine, a nonprofit organization that helps low-income and homeless families. She lived there with her partner assisting troubled and struggling people until her death.

In the lab, things were going well. Our theory of the basal ganglia was drawing a lot of interest from experts in movement disorders around the world. We were frequently asked to lecture in symposia – Jack usually spoke on Parkinson's, I spoke on Huntington's and both of us delivered lectures on the basal ganglia. Our lab had become the most popular among MD/PhD students interested in neuroscience (Figure 11.1). We had a bevy of young men and a handful of women. I was definitely gender-biased. I found it much easier to talk with the male graduate students about their experiments than the females. The guys all said they wanted to make new discoveries about the brain and were passionate about it. I don't really know why I had trouble with women. Maybe I didn't recognize their passion. Maybe they conveyed information differently. I think that there was a certain level at which I didn't understand them. This wasn't true of

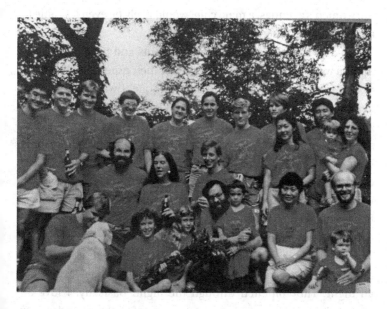

Figure 11.1 Wearing matching T-shirts at our summer lab party in 1990.

Top row from left to right: (unknown), Rich Maciewicz, Brian Ciliax, Zane Hollingsworth, Will Maragos, (unknown), John McDonald, Wake McNeel and Jang-Ho Cha. Middle row from left to right: Jack, me, Jim Olson, Sharin Sakurai and Dorene Markle (and child). Bottom row from left to right: Tony Kincaid, Jessie, Ellen, Roger Albin with son, (Su-Yin) and Tim Greenamyre with son.

everyone, but at that time I think I was so used to dealing with men professionally that when it came to women I was confused. In Michigan, the women's agenda often seemed different than the guys' and they seemed afraid to talk to me. I did my best to treat all of them the same, but I don't know if I really did. It wasn't until later in my career as chief that I learned how important it was to recognize and support women colleagues and mentees. I also learned that unlike men, women don't ask for resources and increased salary. I had to teach them to speak up for themselves. Perhaps I should have known that if I was having trouble relating to the women's agendas, a male chief would likely be even less able to appreciate their talent.

I met with each of the graduate students and postdocs several times a week and went over the plans for their experiments and the results from the ones they had already done. I was fairly good at helping them design the next steps. Jack was shy and wouldn't go and hang around the lab just to see what was going on. The students knew, however, that Jack understood the anatomy of the brain very well. If they asked, Jack would take time and show them the details, but otherwise he was absorbed in his own projects. Jack was also best at data analysis and statistics. For lab meetings, however, he was the one to go out and get the soft drinks and chips. You could always count on Jack for food.

Basically, our lab rocked. We had a loud stereo system that the students turned up full blast when they worked in the lab all night. They pipetted through the night. Basically, I love all my students and would go to the mat for them under any circumstances. I feel as if they are a part of my family. Jack did too. We had frequent lab parties and picnics where we frolicked and played until the wee hours. Our students became our best friends. We did our best to teach them the way to get grants and how to use the system to get their work done and be treated fairly. We promoted them as much as possible to the rest of the scientific world. We were then and I am now incredibly proud of our students and postdocs.

The longer Jack and I lived together, the more we basically became one person. Neither of us were completely independent of the other. We woke up together in the morning and had sex before the kids came upstairs to crawl into bed. Jack read to them while I showered. Then I read to them while Jack showered. We always had breakfast together. We rode our bikes to work and then went to our offices which were right next to each other. We didn't have any independent activities like sports or book groups. We exercised together, shopped together and took the garbage to the dump together. Everything. AnneandJack. JackandAnne.

Both Jack and I thrived on our patients and our colleagues in Ann Arbor. We had developed a multidisciplinary outpatient unit with a nurse practitioner, a speech and language therapist and a psychiatric liaison. Our patients and their families had become part of our lives. We tried our best to keep them well, but the diseases that we treated were irreversible and the patients eventually died. They and we formed a partnership, which was probably why our patients almost always enthusiastically agreed to give their brains for research when they died. Our research depended on them, but our research also depended on our ability to improve their well-being. We could usually help the day-to-day quality of their lives, but when they approached death, they gave their tissues and bodies for research.

Outpatient care of persons with Parkinson's and Huntington's diseases was challenging. In the case of Parkinson's disease, there was a panoply of medications that forestalled the decline and we learned to juggle these judiciously over years. Every once in a while, the medications themselves caused havoc.

A patient of mine, a retired executive with Parkinson's disease, was taking moderate doses of medications for his Parkinson's symptoms. These medications can each cause hallucinations as a side effect. Unfortunately, this man hallucinated that I had told him to stop all his medications. Twenty-four hours after he followed those hallucinations, he took a bath and could not get out of the tub. When his wife came in to help him, he told her that he was fine and that he would soon be out of the bathtub, but he still didn't get up. Despite this seeming emergency, his wife believed him. Twenty-four hours after that, he was still in the tub and stiffer than ever because of his total lack of medication. His wife then finally called the emergency medical services unit which brought him to the hospital. By then, he was so stiff that one person could pick up his head and another pick up his heels and his body wouldn't bend. It took a week to get him back on his medicines and on his feet.

As HD worsened, patients lost their ability to speak clearly. That loss could also cause unintended consequences. One woman I had followed for years had 12 children. The patient and her husband came in one day for an appointment and he said his wife was having outbursts every night after dinner. He didn't know why she became so agitated, but he wondered whether he should give her a sedative at dinner. That sounded like an obvious solution to the problem, but I needed to know what was happening from the patient's perspective before prescribing a sedative. I then spent half an hour simply trying to talk to the woman. After slowly getting words from her, I learned that she became angry every night when nobody cleared the table and cleaned up the dishes! No medicine was necessary. The family just had to set up a schedule for dish washing and things improved on their own.

Roger Albin, Jack and I put together a manuscript titled, "The Functional Anatomy of Basal Ganglia Disorders" as a speculative review for the journal *Trends in Neuroscience* that was published in 1989. The paper examined the existing data from animals and humans. We put the data into circuit paradigms for Parkinson's and Huntington's diseases. The model provided an explanation of the symptoms of Parkinson's disease and the involuntary movements of Huntington's disease. It explained the effects of various neurotransmitters and drugs on the circuits. The model predicted that lesions of the subthalamic nucleus would help Parkinson's disease. Our review was accepted for publication and became our most widely cited paper ever. Our model of basal ganglia function has been challenged by many, many groups, which, of course, was its purpose. Most amazing is that the model has stood the test of time and continues to be cited often 35 years after it was published.

12

• • • • •

The Boat Trip, April 4, 1985

I went back to Venezuela and Lagunetas in 1982 and annually for all subsequent years until the project stopped in 2002. In 1983, Nancy invited Jack to go down to Venezuela as part of the team of neurologists. He was so happy to participate in the project and he became a key investigator who focused on examining the clinical data collected from the patients.

Amazingly, in the spring of 1983, just two years after starting the DNA collecting project, Jim Gusella and his genetics lab at Mass General found a marker that tracked with the HD gene in every affected member of the Venezuelan HD family. The marker was located near the HD gene at the tip of the short arm of human chromosome 4. All humans have 46 chromosomes (22 pairs and two sex chromosomes – one from each parent). This discovery was incredible and happened so quickly! The marker homed in on the locus of the gene on one of our 46 chromosomes. This discovery was the first time the new strategy for gene mapping – what would become the Human Genome Project – had located a novel gene. Now that same approach could be used for mapping other diseases and, indeed, the entire human genome. The discovery made the front page of the *New York Times*, and a news conference took place in the Ether Dome at Mass General. I was invited to attend as one of the study neurologists. It was my first visit to Mass General. It was a giddy time, and we all hoped the actual gene would be discovered soon. Nancy and I rejoiced together. In just three years, she and I had become fast friends, talking frequently about science but also about our personal lives. An avid swimmer and snorkeler, the year after the Ether Dome conference, she visited Jack and me in the Bahamas.

Now the challenge became finding the actual gene involved in Huntington's disease and the mutation causing the disease. The next goal for the Venezuela team was to identify as many new HD cases as possible from the youngest to the oldest age of onset. With every new patient diagnosis, there was the chance of getting closer to the actual gene.

At the basic science level, Nancy, David Housman and MIT Nobel Prize winner Robert Horvitz invited six laboratories with diverse areas of expertise to form a collaborative group to locate the actual HD gene defect as soon as possible. Nancy and the Hereditary Disease Foundation (HDF) provided support for certain key experiments and also brought the group together at least twice a year to discuss progress and exchange methods.

Jack was involved not only in HD research but also in Parkinson's studies. In 1985, he and Ira Shoulson started the Parkinson Study Group. The goal was to have trained investigators at multiple sites who could recruit patients to clinical trials quickly, efficiently and using common evaluation scales. Dozens of institutions joined the effort. The group still exists today. Ira and Jack formed an effective executive team and launched numerous multisite clinical trials on new experimental therapeutics. By having multisite groups all staged and ready to go, a trial could be launched quickly; the approach cut months to years off drug development. Jack participated in the trials by recruiting his patients for the studies.

For Venezuela, Jack was a data man. He loved computers, and because he had taken a course in 'Basic,' he fancied himself a data manager and statistician. He created a database that he wrote himself after his first trip to Venezuela and had our secretary enter all the data after each year's trip. Each year, the amount of data multiplied, in part because Nancy had multiple neurologists examine each patient. I don't know why she did this. Perhaps it was to keep us busy while all the patients underwent extensive neuropsychology examinations. Perhaps it was to get a wide range of opinions that she could choose from. Perhaps it was just to get good data. She could actually examine the patients herself and, in fact, did at the end of the yearly trip when often there were no neurologists left on the team. None of the neurologists except Diana Rosas spoke Spanish as well as Nancy, who based her opinion on the patients' psychological profile as much as their examination – she proved correct more often than we neurologists did.

The database that Jack made, however, was the first complete database of examinations done in Venezuela, and soon it was used to decide who we should see each year. We wrote several papers based on the neurological information and wanted to apply it to the other data, but we did not have the manpower or the knowledge to do that part of the study. One of the first things Jack and I noted in the clinical data was that there were two different clusters of symptoms that progressed over the course of the illness. The first cluster of symptoms to develop were slowness of finger-tapping, slowness of moving eyes from side to side and the amount of chorea, which are irregular dance-like movements. The second symptom cluster consisted of stiffness, tremor and dystonia – not unlike Parkinson's disease. The first cluster developed earlier than the second over the course of the illness. Jack and I realized that the symptom progression was paralleled by the respective loss of first the indirect GABA/enkephalin cells and then later the direct GABA/substance P pathway that we had studied in postmortem human HD brains with Roger Albin and Anton Reiner. In other words, the symptom clusters made sense with and even supported our model.

As personal computers became more powerful and improved software was developed, Jack wrote programs to import the data into more powerful databases. The entry process, however, became more and more difficult as soon we had several thousand examinations to enter each year. Our secretary didn't have time to do it, so we hired work-study students or HD patients to enter it for us.

Every year, Jack and Nancy perused the data and argued about age of onset, diagnosis and progression. Nancy finally tried to 'clean' the data by having it all reentered. Then she talked to Jack about how to decide the age of onset, particularly when two neurologists had different diagnostic opinions. Nancy wanted the data to be perfect and 'scrubbed.' In the last email that Jack wrote to Nancy, he said, "Just don't scrub out reality."

For the most part, Jack and I went down to Venezuela at separate times so as to always have one of us at home with the kids and Joan. The trips were usually for the months of March and April which were hot but fairly dry. Twice we brought our kids down with us – once as little girls when they stayed in the hotel with Nancy's two assistants while we went out and worked. The other time, they were teenagers and came to work with us and took videotapes and photographs of the patients and measured height, weight, handedness and baldness.

In early April 1985, I went without Jack on what started out to be a typical Lagunetas trip. Three people from *NOVA*, the popular PBS science show, joined the trip to film part of a documentary. We headed out around 9 a.m. from Maracaibo going south down the lake in a loaded-up Lagoven diesel-powered boat with its own crew. The boat, loaned to us by the Lagoven oil company, was a big improvement from the Coast Guard boat. Off we went under the bridge and then past San Luis before the coastline gradually receded to our right. It was very hot and humid in the sun, but the wind eased the stifling oppression. I doled out the motion sickness pills. The last thing we needed were seasick passengers. We passed by defunct oil wells and eventually arrived in a forest of active oil rigs, dark and hot against the horizon. Passing close to several, we could see the oil workers sweating in the 100-degree heat and humidity. After five hours, the coastline reappeared, and we eventually recognized the small gap in the coastline.

We arrived near the lagoon, which we had to enter through the narrow opening to get to the town of Lagunetas. We couldn't get in because the water was shallow and a sandbar was in the way. After several hours and numerous unsuccessful attempts, we went down the lake past the opening. There was another entrance just beyond the town, but it was impenetrable too. So, we went down even further, past San Isidro, a little group of houses south of Lagunetas. When we got into the lagoon, the boat ran aground. The captain said, "Sorry, we're just going to have to unpack it here and anchor our boat." It was 6 p.m. and it was starting to get dark. We should have had a pause after this little setback that suggested the crew were not the most knowledgeable or experienced.

But it had already been a long day, and we were eager to get to the houses and set up our equipment and hammocks. We unloaded the boat and put half the supplies in the fishermen's *chalanas*. They took the supplies into the town and would return for the rest of our stuff and for Nancy and me.

"Well, we have to anchor the boat," the crew said. The fishermen went up to the front of the boat and took off the metal cover where the anchor was stored. There it was sitting at the bottom of the chamber. It was dirty and rusted. The crew put the lid back on and wondered what to do next.

I said to Nancy, "What did they just say?"

"They said the anchor is no good."

"What do you mean the anchor is no good? It looks fine."

The crew steered the boat over to an island with some trees on it.

"They are going to try to tie it up to a small tree on the shore, this huge 50-foot boat?" I was aghast. What was the matter with the anchor? Nothing.

Nancy and I opened the cover again and I looked down inside. True, the anchor was bolted in but one of the bolts was rusted out and the other was loose. The anchor hadn't been used in so long that its chain had corroded from the salt. I didn't understand why the crew weren't even going to try to free it, so I went down into the hole and started to chip away at a piece of metal. I finally realized that you could just remove the chain from the anchor and take the anchor out and put it on a rope.

The crew seemed shocked that a woman had gone down in the greasy hole and had succeeded in getting the anchor. One cried, "Que anima!"

We should have realized then that this particular crew was incompetent.

We stayed in Lagunetas for four days, examining, filming and treating the family. We had learned that sleeping in canvas hammocks like the villagers did was the most comfortable way to spend the night rather than sleeping on the nubbly floors. It was one of the hottest stays we had ever had in Lagunetas, with temperatures in the low hundreds and little or no wind. There were rain showers several evenings, and needless to say, the houses leaked and things got soggy. All the ice we had brought had melted by the end of the third day. We examined the family members methodically while the *NOVA* crew taped and interviewed.

On Wednesday, the boat crew came to pick us up. They had taken the boat back to Maracaibo and brought down a new boat.

At noon, the captain said, "Well, the boat's here and we can go any time."

Then we asked him if we had to go now. "Is there any problem? Do we need to go now because of the lake?" We knew in the past that the wind and waves built up on the lake in the evening.

He said, "Oh no, no need to go now."

Nancy had a conversation with him and then I talked to him too. "This is a good boat," he said. The boat had lights and plenty of fuel. "No problema, we can go back at night."

I was surprised. Every other trip, the captain had been anxious about traveling at night because the wind usually picked up then and there were few landmarks to guide the way. This time, the guy said, "No problema." I believed him. We all believed him. It was stupid in retrospect but the desire to stay and finish our work was overwhelming.

Nancy had also asked the captain whether it was possible to go to Congo, a large stilt city on the water about an hour further down the lake. She planned to leave at 5 p.m., go down to Congo, spend a little time, see if there was anyone with HD and then head back to Maracaibo around 7 p.m. Well, we didn't get organized to leave by 5 p.m. It was starting to get dark; the sun was going down and we couldn't have made it to Congo before dark. Thank God we didn't take that little detour. That was probably our only lucky break.

By the time we got out to the boat, Stuart and the *NOVA* crew, who had gone out to the boat earlier, had already drunk a six-pack of beer, maybe even two. Stuart was a bit rowdy. We got the boat packed up. We hauled anchor at around 6 p.m. The sun was six inches from the horizon. As we were heading up the lake into the wind and waves, I started drinking beer too. It had been a productive trip and we all wanted to celebrate. The beer was nice and cold from the ice the crew had brought down that day from Maracaibo. I had had about four beers by 8 p.m., which is when conditions started getting bad. At first, the boat ride was just bouncy, which didn't really bother me, but by 8 p.m. it was so bouncy I could no longer stand on the deck without holding on because with each wave the deck disappeared from under me and then my feet smashed down hard on the deck when the boat came back up. The waves crashed into the bow and washed up over the front windows and sprayed the captain's outpost. The captain was running the boat like a bat out of hell, full blast across the waves.

Nancy asked the captain to slow it down. The waves were getting very big, and I was saying to myself, "Geez! These waves are bigger than I've ever seen here!" We had been out on the lake at night four times before returning from Lagunetas. This time, the lake was rougher than ever; everybody was thrown around. If you didn't stand up and hold on with two hands to something, you could easily be thrown off the deck. So, most of the people were down in the front cabin of the boat where there were seats. The front cabin was about 15 feet long, smaller than the cabins on the other boats we had taken; it was down several steps and had windows in the front just behind the bow. Up the steps, was the captain's perch that looked out over the top of the cabin. The perch was surrounded by windows on three sides and was open to the exposed deck in the back. The long flat metal deck had a railing around it. A big metal chest for ice and supplies was chained to the railing on one side.

Everyone outside stood next to the captain's seat holding on to the railing. Ira had gone down below to sit with his wife, Josie. By this time, the waves were so big that the boat would go down a swell and then come halfway up a swell before the rest of the wave would wash over the bow, crash into all the cabin windows, into the windows in front of the captain's perch, spray over the top and land on the back deck. Even on the back deck we were soaked. Then, all of a sudden, it was like an explosion! This huge crash and whoosh! I was standing at the door of the cabin and I looked down. A huge wave was coming through the cabin. It blew out all the front

214

windows and hit everybody sitting in the cabin full in the face, momentarily covering them. Then, all the water washed down through a false bottom into the bow underneath. Two big waves crashed in, smothering people.

All of a sudden, everyone was racing up the stairs to the deck, coughing up water. The captain slowed the boat. Simon came up first, saying the windows had been totally blown out. I had on a life jacket already, as did Nancy because we had been standing out on the deck. Immediately, the crew went to get the rest of the life jackets. Nelson Marsol, a policeman from San Luis, came up out of the cabin clutching his chest and doing some kind of Hail Mary. He started shaking, saying we were going to die. He asked everyone to pray to San Benito and promise that if we made it out alive, we would all dance to San Benito. Everyone in the cabin panicked. Nancy and I screamed for everyone to calm down. Calm down! It was really scary. The boat was full of water, the waves were just getting bigger and the boat was very close to sinking. Usually six feet above the water, the bow was now just a foot above the water.

The boat was heaving in the waves. Water was still filling up the front cabin where equipment, clothes and hammocks were floating around. There were not enough life jackets. Nancy took off her life jacket and gave it to Nelson. Stuart came up. Stuart the *NOVA* guy. He was plastered. He fell down on the deck. He wanted another beer.

Josie Shoulson's first reaction after getting her bearings was to go down below and start neatening everything up. There were cans of food and bags of clothes floating around in the water which she was picking up and putting in the proper spot. Nelson was doing the same thing. For the first hour, Nelson had just been shaking. He was so scared; he couldn't move or do anything. Simon was the same way. It became clear that cleaning up the cabin wouldn't work because water kept flooding it. Ira found Josie and, together, they just curled up under the captain's seat holding on to each other.

On the other side of the captain's chair, Graciela Penchensahdeh, a colleague from Argentina, started to get violently ill. She got sicker and sicker and sicker. She wanted to jump overboard. We put her in the captain's seat where she could sit comfortably. She was vomiting into a big garbage bag while other people were huddled together, vomiting all over the deck and each other. Everyone tried to find a spot where they could find some safety.

Nancy got out all the hammocks. We found all the clothes we could. I had about three long-sleeved shirts. We put the hammocks and all the clothes on the people who were sick and shivering. As each wave crashed over the deck, you'd get wet and the blowing wind seemed very cold, especially if you were vomiting and dehydrated. Everyone withdrew. Occasionally, Nancy called out some kind of encouragement, but it was brief. I remember looking up at the stars and watching Orion, one of the few constellations Jack had taught me, going around in circles. We were just sitting there, hoping that something would happen. Nothing did.

I think in the first two hours or so everybody thought they were going to die. Then, there were times that things seemed like they were improving, and then they got worse again. I remember having a lot of ups and downs in my own feelings about whether things were going to be okay. Simon said that he was so scared, he just resolved himself to dying. It really got to Ira too.

I was amazed that I didn't have a panic attack and fall to pieces. I guess my adrenaline was going. I had had four beers. I should have been drunk but I wasn't. This was it. If you didn't stay on top of it, you were finished. Nancy was a saint. She was making sure everyone was alive, giving people encouraging little plugs. She is a very strong person. Everyone else was sick as a dog. Ira was incapacitated, puking his guts out. Simon, Maria and Leon had all gotten sick. It was also clear that people had pooped in their pants. Even Steve, who had climbed Mt. Everest and had seen people die, got sick. Nancy didn't sit down for a moment, and she didn't have a life jacket. She had just a T-shirt on. She was standing by the captain's chair helping Graciela. Graciela was so sick she said she wanted to jump overboard because it would be better to die. She felt that throwing up was worse than dying and she was going to die anyway. Nancy was worried but knew it wouldn't happen. I think she was pretty optimistic. She didn't want to sit down with people puking on her. She came over and sat next to me for a few minutes.

I said, "Shit! What a bummer to go down in this!"

"You know, Anne, I don't think anyone is coming to rescue us, but I just don't think we are going to die. We've worked so hard on this project. It's just not destined to be." And she was right.

Though we were out of control, I had my life jacket and I was going to hold on. There were a lot of Styrofoam boxes up on deck and I knew just where they were. They would float. I made sure I knew which one I would use for Nancy. I remember I had my hammock arranged around me so that I wouldn't get caught in it. The ropes were away from my feet. I remember thinking, *I can't get caught in the ropes. If I go overboard, I have my knife, my inhalers for my asthma, and I know where the Styrofoam boxes are.* I knew rationally that our chances of survival were slim. I worried about hypothermia, which was the most likely thing that would have killed us in the lake. After you have been vomiting and braving the waves for that long, you're dehydrated. In the water, the body temperature would gradually cool down toward 80 degrees, which was the temperature of the lake, and we would have ended up dead or near death. If you were fished out and saved, you'd be incoherent. You probably wouldn't remember any of it. You might even survive, but being unconscious in those waves was not good. Many people would have died.

I don't know how long it was, but it seemed like forever. The boat was rolling and pitching, and people were lurching because the waves were huge, up and down on this big roller coaster of continual waves washing over us. The wind was howling, yet it was a crystal-clear night. The stars in the sky were brilliant. I was out on the deck with Steve, and at one point he said, "In all my adventures on mountains, I have never felt so scared and so out of control." The captain tried various strategies to make headway and minimize taking water on board. Every time he tried to go up the lake toward Maracaibo, waves would crash into the cabin and fill it momentarily. There had been so much water taken in that the bow of the boat was actually tipping forward. I knew enough about boats to know that this one had a real good chance of going down. The boat was made out of metal. There were pumps in the aft hold that were always working as long as there was fuel, but the forward hold with all the water had no pump. If enough water had even for a moment gotten into the bow, the weight would shift and the boat would have sunk, just like that.

One of the crew got on the radio and tried calling for help. Nobody answered. Meanwhile, another of the crew found a little portable pump which he jury-rigged with naked wires to power it in the forward hold. We were also trying to bail out. It was a seven-foot bail because we had to get down in the area of the flooded seats and throw the water through the broken windows. Eventually, the bow was lightened enough so that as long as we didn't go into the swells, we would stay afloat. Best was to go along the swells with the waves breaking over the sides of the boat.

The captain finally made radio contact with the oil company. He said that someone would come to get us. I couldn't actually understand all the garbled talk. At one point, Nancy told me that the crew had just asked her to calm people down. They said a helicopter was being sent out. Then they radioed back – no, they couldn't send anyone. Next, they said they were going to send a boat out. At about 11 p.m., they said they couldn't find us and the seas were too heavy to keep looking. They advised us to go with the swells and to try to keep from taking on water. Go to the middle of the lake, not to the side of the lake.

Finally, the crew became seriously worried about running out of gas. If the gas ran out, the pumps would shut down and the electricity would quit, and the boat would sink. The other bad thing was that the swells were getting bigger. As it was, the boat was low in the water and the top of the captain's seat was about eight feet above the water surface. When the boat went down in the trough between the swells, the top of the boat was below the height of the next swell. Even when the boat was going sideways, the waves would swamp the deck. Suddenly, as a swell came over, there was a huge crash! The metal chest that was waist high, six feet long and chained to the railing had been ripped off by a large wave and was careening across the deck and into the railing on the opposite side. It was two feet from me! It was so frightening. By some complete miracle, nobody was crushed by that runaway ice chest. But now the chest was loose. A group of us all grabbed onto it and pushed it off the back of the boat. There were no lifelines. The fact that the big metal chest had been washed overboard confirmed the fact that any of us could have been washed off the deck too.

I then became totally interested in survival. I had my two inhalers and my Swiss army knife in my pockets. If I fell overboard and got tangled in the ropes of my hammock or something, I could cut myself free. I began to plan for all the people without life jackets. I spent those hours thinking about how I would survive. I thought about Jack. I loved him so much. I thought about Ellen and Jessie. I loved them so. They were so smart and imaginative. Their whole lives were ahead of them. Thank God Jack wasn't on the boat – the girls would lose both parents. I hoped that if I died, Jack would find someone nice and kind and comforting to be with. Maybe Nancy would survive and he could marry Nancy. I knew Jack would be a great dad to the girls. He had already proven himself to be more attentive as a parent than I was. He coached their games, went to PTA, ferried them around to parties and friends' houses and he read to them constantly. He never got mad at them and always patiently helped them with their homework. Better me to die than him.

Then we started to head toward the middle of the lake, and about an hour later, we saw a clear light on the horizon. We started going toward it. It seemed so close, but it was one of those horrendously deceptive things. After an hour, we still weren't any nearer. After another hour, we could tell we were getting closer, but it was still faraway. The blinking light turned out to belong to an enormous rig out in the middle of the lake. It was so big; we had seen it blinking from miles and miles away. A huge propane gas rig. We came in slowly. As soon as we saw the light, we had hope. Everybody had some hope. But that optimism faded when we realized that it was also really dangerous. Only a skeleton crew of four people with essentially no amenities manned the rig. They'd flown out to the rig by helicopter and landed on a pad way out on a metal extender arm. The staff on the rig said that we had to make sure nothing could spark because the rig could blow up. Propane gas rigs only had a minimal crew for 24-hour shifts. The crew didn't sleep on the rigs. The guys running our boat didn't want to go near the rig, but Nancy told them, "You're going in there because everyone is incapacitated. The boat is running out of fuel, and we have no alternative except to drown!"

We got the hammocks and draped them over the metal bow and side of the boat. There were several tires we could hang over the side as well. The three or four guys on the rig came down to the landing and threw all the tires they could find over the edge of the platform. Nobody was to smoke cigarettes. The pump in the forward hold that was rigged with bare wires had to be disconnected. Slowly, we approached the rig. It was a rough docking. The crew guys threw the ropes around the pilings and held on as tight as they could, but the boat still lurched up and down. Nancy and I helped steady people as they prepared to jump to the platform. The crew on the rig caught each person and pulled them away from the boat.

Everyone was feeling so sick it was hard to get situated onto the platform safely. The boat was heaving anywhere from four feet below to four feet above the platform. It had to be timed perfectly. We were lucky someone wasn't crushed. As people left the boat, it became lighter and floated higher in the water. The *NOVA* crew kept insisting they had to retrieve their film. Nancy said we had to get the boat away from the platform because the risk of sparks was too high. If we were going to leave our precious blood and skin samples on the boat, then they could leave their film on the boat. They relented and turned to climb up to a higher spot. Then we brought the blood and skin samples onto the platform. By the time the crew pulled the boat away, half the tires were shredded but nothing had sparked.

The propane gas rig was gigantic; it must have been two square city blocks of metal with little catwalks all over it (Figure 12.1). One of the happiest experiences of my life was getting onto that propane gas rig and being on something solid. I wasn't going down in the drink and the chance of the propane rig blowing up was much less than the boat going down. I had tried to be controlled and rational on the boat because that was the only chance I had for survival, but I had also been petrified. On the gas rig, I realized I was completely out of energy. Thank God we're alive! I collapsed and started to cry. I felt awful. I had made it through the whole thing and then I let down and sobbed. Nobody else was crying. I guess if you're that sick you just don't cry. Maybe I didn't notice anybody else crying because it was dark and the rig was unlit. All I could see were huddling shadows. Some people were beyond crying.

The only room on the propane gas rig where you could sit or lie on a floor was a little luncheonette. The rig guys tried to do whatever they could for us. They actually couldn't believe we had made it from Lagunetas – nearly on the other side of the lake. One of the guys said, "I've worked on this rig for fifteen years and God must have blessed your project because I've never seen a boat make it in

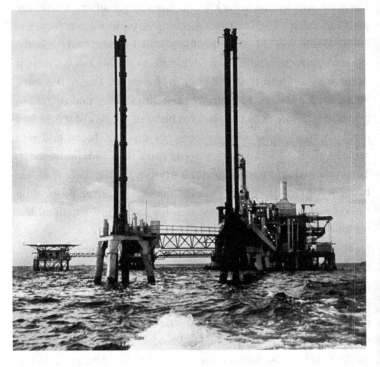

Figure 12.1 Propane gas rig we landed on at 2 a.m.

Unlike oil rigs that have sleeping and eating quarters, propane gas rigs are manned for short stays with a skeleton crew of only four.

weather like this and I've seen many boats go down and many people drowned." He said we were extremely lucky. That drove it home. Everyone found a little space and tried to sleep. We were all still wet and had the continual sense that we were rocking.

One team member actually managed to phone his family in Maracaibo from the rig. He asked them to contact other people and tell them we were safe. His family called Simon Starosta's wife in Ann Arbor who, in turn, called Jack. It was the crack of dawn when Jack got the call. He was all packed and ready to go to the airport because he was coming to Venezuela that day. Simon's wife said, "I just got the message not to worry. Everything's going to be okay." Jack hadn't a clue what she was talking about but had to ponder the mystery all the way to Maracaibo.

The whole thing was so incredible. On the propane gas rig, I remembered wondering during the journey why we weren't seeing any of the smaller, abandoned oil wells, the small square cement structures over a previously active well. They had no lights on them, and I worried that we could have crashed into one. Usually, they were all over the place. When we woke up the next morning, as far as you could see, there was a forest of abandoned wells. I hadn't seen any of them. Thank God I didn't know they were there. I would have been petrified knowing we were weaving through such an obstacle course.

The next day, the oil company sent a replacement boat. Ira got sick again. I wasn't sick so I could help transfer all our gear to the new boat. We loaded up all the puke-laden hammocks into a big pile. The lake was still wavy but not nearly as bad as the night before. Nobody panicked. Nobody was petrified of the boat. Even Graciela who was the most prone to getting sick was okay with getting back on. Nancy said that we were very close to the other side of the lake. We had the choice of going straight to the nearest port and the oil company would pick us up with a bus or we could take the boat on a six-hour trip up the lake. Needless to say, we chose the bus.

When we got to land, we were an exhausted and scruffy group. Ira was wearing a T-shirt, underpants and shoes but no socks. Josie was wrapped in a sheet. Everybody was windblown and soggy. A short royal-blue bus arrived, about half the length of a school bus. We piled the filthy clothes and hammocks in the back and climbed in. Man! Was it great to be on land!

We tootled around the lake in the little blue bus and arrived at the Hotel del Lago at about 5 p.m. on Saturday evening just as all the elite of Maracaibo arrived for dinner and a concert – the men were dressed in their silk suits, flashy ties and slick hair – the women in four-inch spike heels, tight pants, swervy butts, long dark hair and heavy makeup.

The little blue bus came up to the front door and our smelly group staggered out. The people in the lobby stepped to the side like waters parting. We walked through the fancy lobby with our *caritos* (luggage carts) piled with filthy hammocks. It was an unforgettable scene.

Up on the floors, maids rushed to help us. When they heard the story, they were so elated that we survived, they hugged us and immediately rushed all the clothes and hammocks down to the laundry. Within two hours, they brought the clothes and things back, all clean and neatly folded (Figure 12.2).

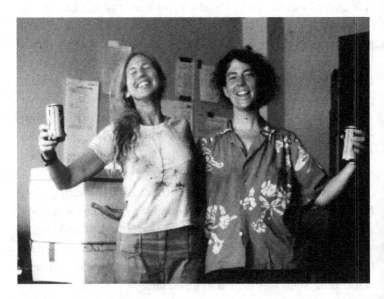

Figure 12.2 Nancy and me celebrating just after arriving safely at the hotel.

Jack arrived later in the evening, and I was so glad to see him after our ordeal. We all spent the evening telling him what happened and how terrified we'd been. We celebrated our survival and promised to dance to San Benito for saving us.

The next day, as we were trying to come to grips with what we had been through, we discussed whether we should go as planned to Caracas to give talks at the university and then on to visit Angel Falls. We had arranged this several months before, and we had all been excited about the possibility of spending four days in other parts of the country. After what had happened, however, we all had second thoughts. Simon Starosta had arranged the lectures at the University of Caracas and his family was going to host Nancy, Jack, Maria Ramos and me for dinner and the night after, and then the next day we were to take off for Angel Falls. In the morning, we decided to bag the trip. We were all wiped out and still frightened.

But over the course of the day, we began to say to one another: "What the hell? Why not? What else are we going to do? Don't we deserve a break?" After all, we had just lived through this ordeal. What else could be worse?

We got on the plane to Caracas. Caracas was a far cry from Maracaibo, tucked into a beautiful valley surrounded by mountains that reminded me very much of California. Caracas wasn't as hot or humid as Maracaibo and had an interesting mix of European culture with elegant buildings from the 1500s and poverty-stricken flimsy tin and plywood houses packed and perched along the surrounding steep hillsides. The city was bustling, but we had little time to see the sights. We went to the university and Nancy and Jack gave talks. Jack had translated his talk into Spanish with the help of a friend of ours and the students and faculty really appreciated his efforts. When it came time for questions, however, he was unable to understand most of them. Fortunately, a few bilinguals helped out.

Chatting with several of the faculty, it was distressing to see how frustrating it was to conduct research in a developing country.

Equipment was sparse and outdated, but worst of all, just getting any supplies or chemicals from the US or Europe was completely unpredictable. For no reason at all, things got held up in customs and sat in hot warehouses only to be released months later when they had degraded or become contaminated. Universities went on strike constantly, so scientists and students might be left suddenly in limbo for weeks or months several times a year. Students often took eight years to get through college or medical school. It was no wonder that talented scientists would do anything to flee such situations.

Things were a bit different for clinicians. Caracas had communities of considerable wealth, and private clinics and hospitals provided state-of-the-art diagnosis and treatment for the rich. Physicians could make a pretty penny in private practice. Working in the university, however, brought only a token salary that nobody could survive on independently, so all physicians worked at least half-time in private practice. Simon's father had been the most prestigious cardiologist in Caracas and his family was well-off. They had a beautiful white stucco house with a traditional Spanish brick style tiled roof. Flowering ivy crept up the outside walls that surrounded the house, and inside the walls the garden was lush and sweet. Glass shards decorated the tops of the walls. Locks on all gates, doors and windows were essential because the crime rates were very high.

The economic difference between the poor and the wealthy was enormous. I was once at a party at the American consul house in Maracaibo talking to an American woman who'd married a Venezuelan and had lived there for years.

I asked her: "Is the consul's house upper class?"

"It's only middle class."

"Who do you consider the poor?"

"The poor are the house cleaners, janitors and garbage men."

"What about the people living on the lake who we were studying?"

She thought for a moment. "Well, they have no class. They get no resources, and they pay no taxes. They just don't count."

The day after staying at Simon's house, we left for Angel Falls. We flew from Caracas to Puerto Ordaz and then switched to a DC9 for the trip to Canaima, the nearest stop to Angel Falls. It was actually the wrong time of year to go up to Angel Falls itself, and besides, it was a week-long hike. But we had been told that the beauty was in the jungle, the Rio Negro and the *tepuis* (jungle-covered mesas) and that Angel Falls was just one of hundreds cascading from the tops of the tepuis.

It was a gorgeous, crystal-clear day, and soon after taking off, we began to fly over jungle. We saw irregularities in the jungle carpet that became larger and larger the farther we went. These were the *tepuis* with vertical walls and flat tops. The pilot said that the jungle species that lived on the tops of the *tepuis* were unique because they had evolved separately in the isolated environment. Jimmy Angel, an American bush pilot and adventurer, had flown over the area many times and had seen the magnificent waterfalls. On one of these trips, he crashed on the top of one of the *tepuis*. By sheer guts and luck, he was able to get down alive, but his wrecked plane could still be seen.

As we looked out the windows, we saw that the *tepuis* were very high and were getting closer together, forming canyons where large rivers ran. The pilot got on the intercom and said in Spanish, "Well, it is such a beautiful day today, we will be able to get a close look at Angel Falls and the surrounding area. Don't worry as we descend. This is completely normal procedure." The plane began to descend and soon we were flying at about 500 feet above the top of one of the *tepuis*. "There is Jimmy Angel's wrecked plane!" the pilot exclaimed. Sure enough, there it was, just below us. We were close enough to see clearly the irregular jungle-covered rock surface of the flat-topped peaks.

Then suddenly, as we reached the edge of the *tepuis*, the pilot rapidly descended over the edge and down into the canyon beside

227

the vertical walls of the *tepuis*. I was on a jet flying through a canyon! Yikes! I held on to Jack but he had leapt from his seat with the camera and went to the other side of the plane to take pictures as we flew by Angel Falls. I followed him. After all, I had no control over what was happening, and it was unbelievably spectacular! All along the near vertical walls of the *tepuis*, waterfalls cascaded down and ultimately landed in the jungle along the edge of the river. Colorful birds flew along the walls below us. The river appeared clear, but it was the color of a dark tea. Tall trees, many blooming, covered the ground.

Down the canyon we went and came out in a valley that was clear of trees. A single long runway greeted us. There was no airport per se. Just a straw-roofed open-air shelter near the runway. There didn't appear to be any town either but that was no problem. Several golf carts came to pick up the passengers and take us to the hotel. It turned out that there was only one resort there – all by

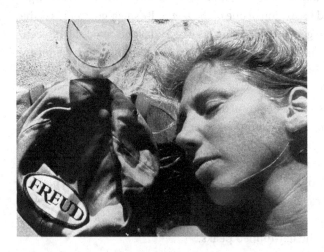

Figure 12.3 Nancy napping on the beach in Canaima, Venezuela near Angel Falls.

itself, just below the beautiful tall but broad waterfalls of Canaima. These falls were several hundred yards wide and divided in the middle by a rock face. They were about 200 feet tall, and they landed in a deep broad pool large enough for boats. Along the edge, was a fine sandy beach. The hotel was a central, open structure for eating and the rooms were in little cabins along the edge of the river. Each cabin had two rooms. Jack and I stayed in one and Nancy and Maria in the other.

Nancy, Maria and I were all wiped out, so Jack said he'd take care of us while we relaxed. We went down to the beach to lie in the sun. Jack bought us piña coladas and then went off to explore the hotel and the possibilities for tours the next day. He came back with plenty of maps and pamphlets. He found out that the resort was run by a couple of Germans who had lived in Venezuela for 15 years.

We took a nap on the beach and then went swimming (Figure 12.3). The water was dark but clear and tasted like tea. We were told that no piranhas lived in the river because of the high tannic acid level. There were fish, however, but not scary ones. When Nancy got out of the water, her blonde hair had been dyed to a tea color! We had a fascinating time going up the river in dugout canoes to islands covered in orchids and bromeliads, swimming holes and beautiful waterfalls cascading down from the tops of the *tepuis*. We returned to Maracaibo rested and ready to take on more long days of work.

13
• • • •

Adventures in Peru

In the years after the discovery of the marker at the tip of chromosome 4, Nancy and her advisors decided on the two most important strategies going forward. First, they put together the collaborative group of laboratories with different genetic technologies to share information and discover the HD genetic mutation. Six laboratories examining separate entities – yeast, fruit flies, *C. elegans* (tiny worms) and humans – set out to work together. The second key activity was to see if all or some of the Huntington's families in the rest of the world shared the same gene marker as in the families we'd found in Venezuela. Nancy never stopped pressing forward. She persuaded scientists and clinicians all over the world to work with her. Her main currency was her charisma. Nancy traveled to Africa, Papua New Guinea, China and India to examine and sample HD families. She identified a number of HD families in Spain and on the island of Majorca. Jack, Jessie, Ellen and I came along to examine these latter families, sample their blood for DNA and take skin samples as we had done in Venezuela.

During all these trips, Nancy and I became better and better friends. I trusted her decisions and followed her direction almost unquestioningly. I could feel her drive, and she did what I would have done. And of course she recognized that I was a kindred spirit, even if my people skills were nothing like hers. In Venezuela, the team regarded me as the person who could tell Nancy to stop working before utter exhaustion made us all revolt. Although Nancy could squeeze water from a stone, I was sometimes able to serve as the brakes on her unfailing desire to work on. She could work the whole day without taking a break. A Food Committee formed among us participants made sure to provide lunch, which was typically *pancitos*, sliced cheese, ham and a couple of Styrofoam boxes full of iced drinks.

I had decided early on in Venezuela that Nancy was the boss. I did as she asked me to do. There were a lot of guys on the team whose professional attitude could be summarized as "fuck this" – they worked on the project for only one year because they felt that they didn't have enough control. Jack was an exception. In particular, some of the men were pissed that at the beginning of the day Nancy might say: "Oh we're gonna go to a town 25 miles north of the city and examine people there." That meant traveling north to another city and examining all the family members. When we got there, we often learned about three or four more branches of the family living nearby that she wanted to examine. Nancy kept us there until the middle of the night. "You're out of your fucking mind, Nancy. Why don't we start again tomorrow morning?" Of course, we never knew what we were going to discover any day we went out – who the neighbors were, who the cousins were, who didn't show signs until age 80. We found ourselves going all over the place in the middle of the night to these little towns. The goal was to get as much done as possible. That was Nancy. If she called you up, you knew she was going to ask you for something. You didn't know what she was going to ask you to do. It didn't matter, because it was always in service to her unrelenting goal to help people suffering from Huntington's.

Nancy was very persuasive, always wearing a delicious perfume. She walked right up to the guys, making it difficult for them to argue with such a beautiful, convincing woman standing before them. When she walked into a room, everyone took notice. She and Marjorie Guthrie, folk singer Woody Guthrie's wife, both had tremendous charisma. After Woody became afflicted with Huntington's, Marjorie became a very active advocate of HD research. She and Nancy both worked on a big commission on Huntington's disease at the National Institutes of Health and Marjorie visited every researcher to say, "Go faster, go harder." I loved Nancy and was grateful for how many times she had saved me and my children when we were in a difficult emotional spot. I would do anything to support her and her work. Besides, I was thrilled to have the chance to meet so many new people and visit so many foreign countries.

Despite our reservations, Jack and I managed to go down to Venezuela together without the kids on a couple of occasions. In 1986, we arranged to both go down together because Halley's comet was going to be especially visible in a remote region like Lagunetas where the ambient light at night was essentially nil.

Jack had it all timed, his binoculars ready. Before he even got up, though, we could hear the men in the town calling out "La cometa!"

How they learned about the comet, I do not know. But it was amazing.

Nancy, Jack and I discussed getting medical support for the family. Jack and I started a foundation for the Venezuelans – the Venezuela HD Family Foundation (VHDFF) – a tax-exempt organization. We found a wonderful woman, Margot DeYoung, who had gone through medical school in her forties and now wanted a job as a generalist. We hired her to work full time year-round for the family. The VHDFF helped with her salary and the Hereditary Disease Foundation helped support her also. She became a saint taking care of the HD families all year long. Eventually, she and Nancy were able to arrange for a hospital to be built in San Luis for the care of the HD patients – Casa Hogar Amor y Fe. The hospital staff were all members of the HD families and so were very familiar with the course of the disease.

Nancy had been in touch with neurologists in Peru in 1985 who said they knew of several large HD families living in a valley several hours south of Lima. Could they be related to the Venezuela family? Nancy wanted to examine them. She arranged for all of us to go to Peru around Christmas time of that year. Jack had recovered well after his bleeding ulcers and now was really game to go on this trip, especially as he had worked in the laboratory at Hopkins with Dr. Tito Arregui, a neurologist who now lived and practiced in Lima. Tito helped us arrange a trip to Machu Picchu for after we finished our work with the HD families. Jack's first trip to Venezuela had been in 1983 and so he was already considered a veteran. Nancy had, in fact, gotten all the veteran people on the Venezuela trip to come along on this Peru trip. Graciela Penschensadeh (an Argentinian), Maria Ramos (a Spanish geneticist), Ira Shoulson, Fidela Gomez (an Argentinian nurse) and us. It was to be a New Year's vacation, and we bought plane tickets for all of us to leave on December 20th and return in early January. Jessie was eight and Ellen was six. We thought that people in Peru were less impoverished than the people we had found in Venezuela and imagined the trip with the girls would be safer. I don't know where we got this idea, but once we got on our way, we found out we were wrong.

We arrived in Lima in the middle of the night and Dr. Cuba (the Lima neurologist who knew the HD families) met us at the airport and took us to the Hilton Hotel. It was a beautiful hotel and clearly one of the ritziest in the city. The next day, we visited with Tito and then we rented two Toyota pickup trucks, each with two seats and an open flatbed. As soon as the Peruvian medical students, who had volunteered to go with us on our trip to examine the families, saw the trucks they gasped in dismay and told us that they would have to ride in the back on top of all our bags and supplies because otherwise they said our luggage would be stolen off the backs of the trucks while we were driving. We were startled. How could they take things if we were driving on the highway? Simple, they said. Another pickup truck just gets going the same speed as you and one of two men jumps from his truck to yours and starts tossing the bags into the other truck. It was one of the more common modes of theft.

Lima was hot, dry, and covered in a layer of soot that gave a dark and sinister feel to every street and park. There were almost no green trees. Dr. Cuba took Nancy and us to the hospital where he worked. He looked after patients in a large neurology ward. The ward was in a solitary, whitewashed, blue-trimmed building with its own entrance. Inside, it was also painted blue and white. The long room was filled with beds lining each side – about 50 beds in all. Most patients had been there for prolonged stays of weeks, months and even years. Jessie and Ellen had come along. Jessie stayed a good distance away from the patients, but Ellen kept close to the doctor as we went from bed to bed. Torsion dystonia, severe head injury, Friedreich's ataxia ... on down a litany of illnesses. From time to time, Dr. Cuba pulled back the sheet covering a patient and Ellen's eyes (which were just about on a level with the sheet) opened wide in horror as she saw the crooked limbs underneath.

Later that first day, we went over to Dr. Cuba's house away from downtown Lima. A gated entrance accessed the property which was surrounded by a wall topped with glass shards. His home inside the walls was open and bright with marble floors and floor-to-ceiling windows looking out over a large, green lawn and garden. Jessie and Ellen played in the yard while we sat on a stone terrace in the sun having iced tea.

The next day, we loaded up our trucks with bags and supplies despite the risk of theft, and the medical students sat on top of the luggage to deter any robbers. We started down the highway south along the coast. After two to three hours, we came to Cañété at the mouth of a river valley on the coast. We wanted to get hotel rooms in the city so we could drive up the valley during the days to examine and sample patients. The city had a hotel, but the rooms were singles, with common bathrooms, and there was no hot water. Not quite what we wanted. The medical students contacted Dr. Cuba, but he didn't know of any alternative. They talked to Tito who said he would ask his sister who knew of several additional hotels. Tito's sister said we could take a chance on a hotel up the valley – a four-star hotel aimed at tourists which might have vacant rooms even though it was the holiday season. The only doctor in Cañété agreed and said that it would be a good place to have as a home base because the families lived close to that particular hotel.

We got in the trucks again and headed up the valley. By now, it was midafternoon. We drove on and on, and at about two hours out, the pavement disappeared and the towns and houses were without electricity. Finally, as the sun was setting, we saw a sizable fluorescent sign off to the left that said, "Hotel Embassy." The sign announced a large L-shaped, two-story whitewashed building with two cars out front, both white and old but very swank for Peru and definitely nicer than any we had seen for the past two hours. There was a dim fluorescent light in the green and white office and a man sitting beside the desk. He had a ledger to the side of the desk. The students and Graciela inquired about rooms and the man said, "Oh no! No rooms." He explained he was full up because it was vacation and the holidays.

The students mentioned the name of the person who recommended us and then he seemed to soften up. "How many rooms do you need?'

"Nine – four doubles and five singles." He only had doubles, but the price was more than reasonable.

The rooms were beautiful with normal-size twin beds and nice sheets and bedspreads. Each room had a bathroom and hot water, and we looked out over the Cañété Valley. There was even a pool. The kids were excited about going swimming but then we saw that despite the pool being a beautiful blue-green, it was also as cloudy as milk. Oh well, we were all hungry and descended on the restaurant. I remember the crayfish and rice stew I ate that first night. It was delicious. As far as we could see, there were only two other people staying there even though the manager had said the hotel was full. Maybe it will fill up tomorrow, we thought.

We gave each of the girls a Polaroid camera for Christmas and their job on the trip was to take pictures of people in the HD families and write the person's name on the back. They were just six and eight, but this job kept them engaged most of the day. Jessie was very bright, an excellent reader and she wrote out the person's name on the photographs. Besides, there were plenty of other neurologists and so either Jack or I could take the day off to play with the kids. They almost always wanted to go with the medical team. The experience made a big impression on all of us. Most of the families we were studying were very poor and living in mud-walled huts with dirt floors and without electricity. Unlike the Venezuelans who used hammocks, the Peruvians just slept on the dirt floor. On the other hand, even the littlest kids went to school and could write their name because, unlike Venezuela, the government covered books and uniforms.

We had given Jessie and Ellen origami papers and little books to teach them how to fold things into various shapes. In the evening at the hotel, they figured out how to make a stork or a bird and then

236

show the kids in the village the next day. Everyone seemed delighted to be together and no one had to speak Spanish to communicate with one another.

Politically, the valley was split into those who supported the dictatorship and the Maoists who wanted to overthrow the government. As long as we stuck with the doctor, we were safe since he made his living off both sides. Most of the people had only seen American supporters of the Shining Path. The Shining Path or Sendero Luminoso was a communist, terrorist guerrilla group controlling many of the mountain regions in Peru. A number of Americans had joined the guerrilla group. So once, when Graciela and I walked into a store by ourselves (we were dressed in blue jeans, T-shirts and baseball caps), everybody split because they thought we might rob them.

We spent two weeks going up and down the valley, from town to town and house to house finding, questioning and examining families affected by Huntington's disease. Along the way, we saw beautiful vistas side by side with extreme poverty. Despite desperate conditions, the people were neat and courteous, and they did their best with what little they had. We never had to worry about our physical safety.

We did worry about our tires. They were all bald and one of them blew out on us. Jack and I fixed it, and when we took the bad one in to get it fixed, we asked about new tires. The guys at the store just laughed and said that they would consider the tires we did have *new*. Peru apparently had virtually no new tires except for those brought in personally. That explains the frequent sightings at the airport of people traveling from Miami to many South American countries with shrink-wrapped Michelin tires.

At the hotel, no new guests were showing up. It was past Christmas and New Year's and the place was empty. At the hotel restaurant, there was little food except for dishes with crawfish that the staff had caught down in the riverbed. All the chickens were eaten as were the potatoes. We were getting down to their last Coke and saltine crackers. Ellen basically refused to eat anything except bread and crackers. Obviously, the hotel wasn't used to having so many guests.

The morning before we were going to leave, we asked whether we could pay the hotel in traveler's checks and were told, "Absolutely not. No US dollars. Only intis [the local currency]."

Graciela whispered to me, "Oh. That's it. Why didn't I think of that? Everybody elsewhere in Peru always wants dollars!"

Suddenly, I also realized what was going on. A quick glance at the ledger made it all make sense. The hotel was 'full' of all sorts of imaginary guests paying in dollars. This was a money-laundering operation complete with four-star rooms, restaurant, pool and laundry! To the authorities, the luxury hotel was very 'profitable'; its accounts were totally 'in order' and easily 'brought in' $1,000,000 a year. It wasn't really a hotel; they just had this stage setup. Now and then, a couple here, a couple there. It took little money to run the operation, just a few maids. Because they worked with the drug cartel, their buddies had millions of US dollars from selling drugs that had to be 'accounted' for. The hotel was the perfect front. The ledger indicated the hotel was always completely full of fake guests paying in dollars.

We went down to Cañété and asked the doctor where we should go to change dollars into intis and he said not to go to the bank because if we did everybody in town would know it within minutes and we would never get back to the hotel with the money. When we asked what we could do, he pulled out big wads of bills from his back room and said he would be happy to change our money.

We did as the good doctor instructed and got back to Lima safely without any untoward events or mishaps.

From Lima, Nancy, her boyfriend Herb Pardes, Jack, the girls and I got on a train to go to Cusco and then Machu Picchu. Cusco was a truly amazing high-altitude city mainly occupied by native

Peruvians who were descendants of the Incas. We spent the next day in Cusco and Ellen fainted dead away after breakfast. High altitude or fatigue? The next day we were off to Machu Picchu. As we entered the station, Ellen turned green and started throwing up. Nancy, who hated vomiting, huddled around Ellen to make her feel better but it was really pathetic because Ellen could little afford to throw much up since she hadn't eaten in days. That afternoon and evening in Machu Picchu were spectacular. Jessie came out with us as Ellen recuperated in her room. In keeping with all of it, Jessie got sick the next day and Ellen went out with us.

14

· · · · ·

Being Recruited

I was one of a handful of women in neurology who were truly 'academic' – doing NIH-supported research, teaching students and residents, and seeing and treating neurological patients. As a matter of course, every search committee in the country had to justify to their institution that they had done due diligence in affirmative action and sought out potential female candidates. Thus, in about 1983, I began to get letters of interest from various institutions searching for candidates for tenured positions, professorships or even department chairmanships. In 1990, I received a letter from the Massachusetts General Hospital asking if I would be willing to be a candidate for chair of the Department of Neurology at the hospital and Julieanne Dorn Professor of Neurology at Harvard Medical School.

Since I was happy in Michigan, I usually declined these letters, but this one piqued my interest. The place was supposed to be the pinnacle of traditional, male-dominated medicine. Could they be serious? I knew they had a really strong neuroscience research group that had been assembled by the former chair of the department,

Joseph B. Martin, a neurologist and neuroendocrinologist who had come to Mass General from Canada 12 years earlier and started the Boston Huntington's Disease Center Without Walls in 1978. As part of a grant for the center, Joe had asked MIT geneticist David Housman to write up a project to find the HD gene. Housman had not only written up the project but also suggested that Joe recruit David's graduate student, Jim Gusella, to start the hunt. Jim was the person to whom we had been sending all the Venezuela blood samples over the past nine years. Why not write back that I was interested and send in my CV?

Some months later, when I received a call inviting me to visit, I was very surprised. I couldn't believe my ears. But why *not* visit? I had previously visited Mass General for one grant review and for another visit when the localization of the Huntington's disease gene was announced in 1983. This time I'd be able to really see the hospital close up.

At Logan airport, I was picked up by a Mass General security officer and whisked to the Ritz Hotel. My itinerary lay waiting at the desk. The next morning, a car picked me up at the hotel and took me to the hospital, where I waited in the lobby for my first interview. I had on a shirt dress, low heels and stockings. I wore no makeup and my hair fell in a large ponytail from my right shoulder. I didn't carry a purse – only a soft leather briefcase. There wasn't anything distinctly wrong with my appearance, but I considered myself more casual than a serious job candidate ought to look. I didn't own a power suit with big shoulders as was then in vogue for professional women. I guess others felt the same way because when I approached a woman gazing around the lobby as if she were looking for someone and asked if she was looking for Dr. Young, she seemed surprised when I said I was her.

All day I met with different people every half hour, and then in the late afternoon, I met with the entire search committee in John

Potts' office. Potts was the chief of medicine and the head of the search committee. His spacious office was comfortable and had oriental rugs and several couches. Everyone was very pleasant. When they asked about my goal for the department, I decided to be perfectly frank because I didn't really think they would pursue my candidacy. I was sure that I was just being interviewed to fulfill the search committee's need to look at women and minority candidates.

"Well, the science is very strong," I said. "But the clinical research and excellence can be improved. I consider the best disease-focused neurology team to be one in which there are basic researchers (spending full time in the lab), clinician scientists (spending 80 percent of their time in the lab and 20 percent of their time in the clinic seeing subspecialty patients), clinician investigators (who do clinical research on patients and test potential new drugs) and clinicians (who are the clinical experts seeing patients full time). I want to make the department the best in the world."

When the head of psychiatry asked me what it felt like to be a woman in a male-dominated field, I said that being in a male-dominated field was no big deal for me. I had been lucky to have male mentors who supported me along the way. Fortunately, they were not chauvinists the way many other male colleagues could be. I told him that I just ignored the chauvinists and considered them jerks. I had also met women who acted like jerks. I assured him that I could handle difficult people regardless of gender.

I went home. I kind of liked the people I had met. The position actually intrigued me. I told Jack, which made him a bit nervous. We were so settled in Michigan. Change seemed daunting.

The people at Mass General asked me back for a second visit and then a third. Each time, I liked the institution better. After meeting with their business people, I surmised that opportunities existed in the overall budget to make some easy changes that would improve the patient services and bring in more revenue. Then in late September 1990, I got a call at home from John Potts and he offered me the job. I was shocked. They had seriously chosen me? Wow! Unbelievable! Now I had to think seriously about making a decision. Could I do this? Did I want to? What about Jack and the kids?

Jack and I went outside and had a cigarette and discussed the possibilities. We rarely smoked more than a half a pack of cigarettes a week but we found an occasional smoke relaxing and made it easier to talk. Mass General had one of the best neurology services in the country and I could bargain for a package that could make it *the* best. Boston was near Jack's family, which was a plus even though his mother had died. The girls were about to change schools anyway – Ellen into middle school and Jessie into high school. However, Jack wasn't that keen to leave his patients and his secure position. In order to make the move work, Jack would have to be appointed full professor of neurology at Harvard Medical School and the two of us would have to get nice labs. We figured that we would not take the job unless we got what we wanted in terms of funding, resources and appointments.

Next, I called Nancy, who was amazed and excited by the fact that I was offered the job. She suggested I talk to Herb for advice on how I should respond. Herb was then the dean of Columbia University College of Physicians and Surgeons and had lots of experience recruiting department chairs. He suggested that I write a prospective plan of what I wanted to do if I took the job. Herb, like Milton Wexler, Sid Gilman and others, was part of a group of powerful, assertive, successful men who wanted to see me succeed. I was fortunate they respected me and my work. They were men who knew how to handle power, and I intentionally sought out their advice when I was unsure of how to handle a new and challenging situation. Unlike other women I've met who have also needed the support of older male superiors to advance in their profession, I was lucky that my mentors treated me well and didn't screw me over literally or figuratively.

I put together a five-year plan and had Nancy, Jack and Herb look at it before I sent it to Mass General. Mass General liked the plan and wanted me to put numbers to it. I was aided in this by Jack who developed a detailed Excel spreadsheet that included projected costs for various recruits over a five-year period. When I asked Nancy and Herb for tips in how to best negotiate, Herb said to never beg or whine but rather negotiate as if I were *Columbo* – the detective in a popular TV serial played by Peter Falk. Columbo was a frumpy detective who always had another question to ask when trying to expose the murderer. Scratching his head, playing dumb, he would ask something completely obvious like, "I'm just trying to understand how the knife appeared on your bedside table?" Herb elaborated on this Columbo strategy. "Don't just come out and say you need millions of dollars," he advised. "Show what you want to do to make the department the best in the world and then scratch your head and wonder out loud how you could possibly accomplish that without adequate support. Then conclude you can't."

I couldn't decide what I wanted to do. It was a big decision and my whole life would be changed by this move. Did I want to be a department chair? Sometimes I concluded yes, other times I concluded no. The people in my lab made a thermometer that had a temperature indicator reflecting the likelihood that I would go. It could be raised or lowered at will. I had to make sure Jack would be supported by the department and grants. In addition, I particularly wanted Zane Hollingsworth to come if we moved to Boston. Zane had run my lab for 11 years. He knew all the equipment and experimental protocols. He was level-headed and made a point of being able to obtain *anything*. He and his wife had just finished building a brand-new house in Ann Arbor so I had to make the move appealing to them. Part of my

244

negotiations with Mass General insisted on an excellent salary and position for Zane.

I needed more advice. At the Hereditary Disease Foundation annual workshop and Scientific Advisory Board meeting, held in Santa Monica, Nancy said I should talk to her father, Milton Wexler. Milton was thoughtful and calm and, like Herb, he was also straightforward and to the point. I spent an evening with him discussing the pros and cons of going to Mass General. At the end of the conversation, he summed up his opinion as: "Bargain for what you want and take the job if they give it to you. If they don't, walk away." He said there is always a balance point and if the people making the offer were willing to tip it in my favor, I should take the job. If not, decline. Although simple, it was such good advice and now I had a plan.

I brought my Excel spreadsheets of financials and my written proposal for five years of support to show the hospital leadership. They liked it, and when I met the CFO of Mass General, he took a deep breath and said he'd give me what I had asked for – millions that would cover recruits and expenses for five years. Jack would be appointed professor of neurology and Zane instructor at Harvard Medical School. We would get new renovated labs located next to other productive neuroscientists.

Now the decision was made. When I told Sid, he was sad to lose Jack and me but also proud that two of his 'children' were moving up to such a prestigious department. He offered all his advice to me and encouraged me to talk to his head of finances for the department for more specifics. One thing he said that stuck with me and that I found especially helpful was if faced with a particularly difficult decision, it was effective to invite an outside group of luminaries to consult for and advise you. Well, in a sense, I had done that already with Herb and Milton. More to the point, Sid suggested that when evaluating the excellence of a particular subspecialty, it was effective to invite experts in the specialty from outside institutions who could critique the group's expertise. That way, I could use advice from the outside experts to reshape the unit. And I wouldn't be directly blamed for any unpopular changes the reshaping required. Sid was truly an outstanding mentor and role model, and I promised myself that I would do my best to emulate his open, honest and helpful style.

Telling the girls that we were going to move brought out all their personality differences. Jessie, who was always comfortable with change said, "Hey! That will be fun!" She was confident and independent.

Ellen, on the other hand, had a very different opinion. "Mom, it would just be better if you died. If you die, then Dad won't go. Face it, Mom. You haven't been the greatest mother – you work all the time. My friends go to their mothers if they have problems to solve but you are never around. I realize that you love your work so I just developed close friendships instead and now you are going to take me away from my network of support."

Whoa! Dig it in. Ellen could really put a stake through my heart. Later, after the kids were in bed, Jack and I started laughing. Ellen had always been resistant to change. At least she knew how to speak her mind. I hoped I could make the transition less painful for her.

I began spending one to two days a week in Boston. I met with each of the faculty and with the hospital and department business administrators. I bonded with Jane Holtz, the vice president for the hospital who was in charge of neurology, neurosurgery, neurobiology and psychiatry and she gave me outstanding advice about how to navigate the complex politics of the hospital. I learned when to make a phone call instead of writing a letter. A phone call doesn't leave a written record. I learned when to compromise and when to insist on my decision.

I asked each faculty member what they needed and what concerns they had. They were remarkably quiet. I learned afterwards that several had complained that they didn't feel empowered to communicate with me. I was surprised because nobody had asked for anything. It took a while for me to realize that they were tiptoeing around and trying to read between the lines in what I said. I finally had to tell each person as they came in to meet with me that I couldn't read their minds and that they should ask outright for what they wanted or they wouldn't get it. It was only then that they learned my Midwest forthrightness.

I arranged weekday trips to Boston for each of the girls, and in February, we went house-hunting. As chief I would need a house where we could entertain all the residents twice a year. I fell in love with a classic old colonial in Boston that had had only two owners the last 50 years. It had a wonderful front hall, wood-paneled living room to the left and a big dining room to the right. The living room had French doors that opened to a large, beautiful screened porch. The price was low because it needed a lot of work. I talked to Jack and we decided to buy the house before he had actually seen it. (We did show him pictures.)

My brother-in-law, Paul Cronin, knew a good contractor who was flexible about how he worked. I contemplated getting an architect but, in the end, decided against it and instead the contractor and I worked together. We designed a new kitchen, painted the house, redid all the heat and electrical, and added a bath on the third floor. It was almost done by the time we had to move in. Jack had sold our house and coordinated the movers. Packing the house turned up dozens of 'wah-wahs' (pacifiers) that Ellen had lost over the years.

We said goodbye to Joan, who was no longer living with us but with a nice man who worked as a car mechanic in Ann Arbor.

Neurology is a specialty that involves long-term care for people with various chronic illnesses such as Parkinson's and Huntington's diseases, epilepsy, multiple sclerosis and stroke. We had cared for many of our patients for 13 years and helped manage their illnesses and disability. We were close to a great many of them and their families as well. They were proud that we were going to the Mass General but they were also very sad to see us go. Several patients came to Boston to continue their care.

Both of us cried in the office with the patients in saying goodbye.

To ease the transition, Ellen invited one of her good friends from Ann Arbor to visit shortly after we arrived. Hurricane Bob was barreling along toward the Cape and a direct hit on Boston. Jack and I went into work but went home when the wind whipped up and the rain came down in deluges. I had never seen anything like it. Then the eye of the storm came across followed by another siege of rain and wind. I found the hurricane exciting and was certain that all the tall old trees at the back of our yard would come down. But they remained standing.

15

• • • • •

First Woman Chief at Mass General

In Ann Arbor, the university health system where Jack and I worked was a leading national hospital, but we had little local competition and felt pretty secure that we were the only game in town. In Boston, at Mass General, the stakes were higher and the game was a lot more complex. We were one of six hospitals affiliated with Harvard Medical School and consequently had to compete intensely for faculty, space and resources with the Dana Farber Cancer Hospital, the Beth Israel Hospital, the Boston Children's Hospital, the Brigham and Women's Hospital (Brigham) and the Massachusetts Eye and Ear Hospital. Each hospital had their own leadership, hierarchy and were independently run. All of this set the stage for fierce turf battles, politicking and personality clashes. Because most doctors at the hospitals also had teaching and academic appointments at Harvard Medical School and medical students rotated through each of the hospitals during training, there were also many opportunities for interaction and collaboration.

As department chief I had to work with the hospital's highest echelons. I learned a lot about leadership styles. When I was recruited, the president of the Mass General was Bob Buchanan. He was very formal. Very aloof. He worked behind the scenes to achieve his agenda. That was the way things got done. Everything was a deal but ultimately he called all the shots. At 6'6", he was literally the big cheese. He held forth at the weekly meetings I attended with the other chiefs of service. I was the only woman sitting at the table; other women – administrators and assistants – sat in a back row of chairs. At my first meeting, the man sitting next to me whispered, "Do you feel comfortable here?" I answered, "I did until you asked me."

Buchanan listened to what everyone said and then went ahead and did whatever he wanted. He definitely played favorites – particularly the heads of medicine and surgery. Fortunately, he supported me and seemed to treat me like one of his daughters. In 1993, Buchanan retired and was replaced by Sam Thier, who was then president of Brandeis University. Sam had trained in medicine at the Mass General so he knew the landscape. Sam was a man of action and he was very dedicated to the institution. Although he was lean and could be mean, he was generally very thoughtful, ethical and practical in his approach to problems. He listened to what we all had to say and then used our input to act as he thought best for everyone. I appreciated that, unlike Buchanan, he kept all the chiefs informed of what and where he had decided to do and go.

In addition to Jane Holtz, I was fortunate to inherit Sherri O'Grady, my business manager. Sherri was from Nebraska. She was married with two small sons. In the evening, she attended business school classes and was earning an MBA. Jane had grown up in Boston and obtained her PhD in business administration from Harvard University before joining the staff of Mass General. She had two grown children. Jane and Sherri worked well together although Jane was 20 years Sherri's senior. Because they both felt vulnerable at night in the neighborhood near the hospital, they went together to a shooting range to learn how to shoot handguns and subsequently carried guns in their purses. Sherri and I brainstormed about projects for the department and then she put our ideas into a business plan with the help of Jane who then took it to the president of the hospital. Working as a team, we arranged many proposals for space and resources and were often successful.

When it came to neurology, Mass General was a Boston star. The Mass General Neurology Service was renowned for its extraordinary triumvirate of senior leaders in the field: Raymond D. Adams, C. Miller Fisher and E. P. Richardson. In their eighties, they still came to work daily, taught students and saw patients. They had been among the first to describe many neurological conditions, from alcohol withdrawal to stroke and neuropathology. I was honored to work with them, and they were very welcoming and supportive of me. Their work was their life.

I got a taste of this in October when I decided to attend on the Inpatient Service that month: seeing and examining all the admitted patients and teaching the residents and students. One Sunday morning, when I arrived at the inpatient floor at about 8 a.m., I saw Dr. Miller Fisher sitting at the nurses' station and jotting down notes in a patient's chart.

"Hi Dr. Fisher. Is there anything I can help you with? It's a spectacular fall day. Crisp blue skies with peak fall colors. I hope you and your wife can get out for a drive." My first New England autumn, I was amazed by how beautiful the countryside became when the foliage flamed red, orange and yellow.

"Oh, good morning, Anne. Well, I am just documenting my patient's response to treatment. My patient came in on Friday night with an evolving stroke. I have been treating him with heparin."

"I'm happy to watch your patient today and you can enjoy the outdoors."

"Well, for me, it's critical to watch the patient's response to therapy."

"I can follow the response for you."

"I'm afraid you don't understand. I have been here since Friday night, personally giving the patient heparin every four hours intravenously. I then document the response in the chart."

"You have been here two days since Friday night?"

"Yes. It's my approach to patient care. I learn a lot from each case."

I soon learned that Dr. Fisher was an extraordinarily dedicated physician who personally attended to the patient no matter how long the hours. In World War II, he had been a prisoner of war in Germany. As the most senior officer among his fellow Canadian prisoners, he spent as many hours as possible in the camp commandant's office requesting help for his group. Time had no meaning for him in the war. Time was also unimportant when patients had to be seen. Dr. Fisher was renowned in his knowledge of stroke. His work ethic was also adopted by other faculty.

One adopter of Dr. Fisher's ethic was Walter Koroshetz, who I quickly learned was a superb doctor, teacher and investigator. He had five children, but he spent most of his time in the hospital. I made him head of the residency program and vice chair of the department. He was an expert in stroke and critical care but also saw patients in the HD clinic. In his 'spare' time, he worked in a lab. Basically, he was overcommitted but he loved all the different aspects of his work and tried to keep them going. Eventually, he became part of the team with Jane, Sherri and me.

Walter's clinical skills and dedication to patient care made him a favorite of the residents and other doctors in the hospital. He was available day and night to come into the hospital to assess a patient. In fact, I was impressed early on with the work ethic of most Mass General physicians. At night, there were always faculty in the hospitals with the residents. In 2007, Walter was recruited to the NIH as deputy director of the NINDS. He is now director of the NINDS.

My department had about 200 faculty and trainees (Figure 15.1). I was in charge of all but about 10 people. These 10 people were appointed at the hospital as private practitioners; they were not department members at the mercy of the department chief. Unlike the majority of my faculty, who earned annual salaries based on their grants, patient care and teaching, the private practitioners made their income by seeing as many patients as possible. They were able to do this in part because when their patients were in the

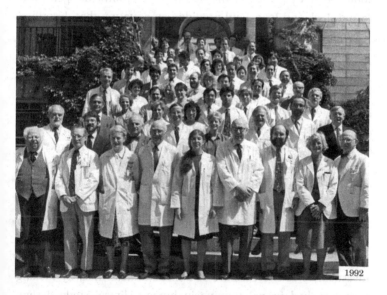

Figure 15.1 Department picture in 1992. Courtesy of Mass General Photography.

Front row (left to right): Mandel Cohen, E. P. Richardson, Tessa Hedley-Whyte, Raymond D. Adams, me, C. Miller Fisher, Jack, Shirley Wray and Steve Parker.

hospital they used the neurology residents, with whom they had no official relationship, as free labor. I made sure to recruit no new private practitioners and gradually the existing ones retired.

Jack loved the fact that our lab was just five floors above the basement neuropathology laboratory. He went to each weekly Brain Cutting Conference where E. P. Richardson, Tessa Hedley-Whyte or Jean-Paul Vonsattel would preside. After hearing the clinical course of the patient's illness, Jack enjoyed trying to guess ahead what the brain would show. Jack also spent hours looking at HD brains with Jean-Paul, who was the world's most experienced HD neuropathologist. The two of them could look at brain sections using the two-headed microscope. They would cruise around the sections both knowing where they were and look for new features of the disease. Later, after the gene was found, Jack and Jean-Paul provided an equation that described the age of onset, severity and disease progression based on the neuropathology, repeat number and age at death from many cases.

I started to build the subspecialty neurology services according to my model I had presented to the search committee. I helped promote the basic scientists and I recruited several clinician scientists to link the researchers to the clinicians. I recruited several clinicians to fill gaps in the services and inherited the makings of several teams where the import of one or two new recruits completed the team. I was also full of optimism for the development of truly new therapies for neurologic disease. In preparation for the time when these studies would begin, I spent most of my start-up funds on recruiting and training clinician investigators in the conduct of human clinical trials by making sure they had formal training in human clinical study design, including informed consent forms, the statistics for analyzing study results and ethical issues associated with clinical trials. Over time, we developed outstanding programs in neuromuscular disease, stroke, movement disorders, memory disorders, epilepsy, behavioral neurology and neurogenetics.

The Mass General had made important contributions to our understanding of stroke. Miller Fisher had described various types of stroke and had innovated interventions aimed at breaking up any blood clot causing a stroke. He had trained stroke experts who now practiced all over the world. At Mass General, he had trained Philip Kistler, Ferdi Buonano, Walter Koroshetz and Daryl Gress. The problem with this team was that each person had substantial patient care responsibilities and no time to actually do clinical research. Adding two postdoctoral fellows to work with them full time gave the team the manpower to see more patients and help run clinical trials. This small amount of added support allowed the Stroke Service to thrive.

In a similar way, I tried to enhance the Epilepsy Service, Behavioral Neurology Service and Movement and Memory Disorders Service. The doctors in the resulting subspecialty service met together to see patients in the outpatient unit. That allowed the specialists to share cases and knowledge and learn from working together. Students, fellows and faculty all saw patients on a given morning or afternoon. As the services grew, additional mornings or afternoons could be added, but we soon ran out of clinic space. Our department had at least 65,000 square feet of research and clinical space. I knew where every neurology square foot was at the hospital. I was always looking for more space. I took advantage of the fact that if our grants were large enough to bring in full 'indirects' (money added to grants to help pay for lights and heat throughout the institution), I could make a compelling argument to Mass General for giving us *more* space.

One big disappointment for me and Jack was that we were not particularly welcome in the Mass General Huntington's outpatient clinic. A diverse group of Mass General doctors saw the HD patients and the clinic provided nutritional, physical and occupational therapy advice for each patient. I suppose we could have joined the group whether they liked it or not but we decided to just see our own HD patients as they made appointments to see us.

That first year, I had to fire my executive assistant because she was racist, impatient, intolerant and very rough around the edges. I couldn't find a replacement. The assistant I had fired knew everybody in the hospital and told everyone I was impossible to work with. Finally, a candidate came to interview who was not from the hospital but from a lab in the big Mass General research facility. She was friendly and outgoing. Beverly Mahfuz. She had grown up and attended school in Lowell, north of Boston.

"Tell me a little about yourself," I said. "I have dyslexia and am a very poor reader. I need help with reading letters and emails. Are you a fast reader?"

"Very fast. I read a couple books each week on the train. I love to read." I took a breath. So far, so good.

I told her that, at 200 people, the department was large and that many trainees and researchers were from countries other than the US. "How do you feel about working with different kinds of people and foreigners?"

"Well, my husband is of Syrian descent and he shops abroad for rugs for his family's business. I also like to travel and enjoy meeting people from different backgrounds."

That was it. Hiring Beverly was the best choice I made after taking over the department. She fit right in with Jane Holtz and Sherri O'Grady and me. She read all my mail and pointed out the things I had to respond to. Her work was impeccable. I trusted her completely and we became friends. Beverly was key to my success. Not only did she know what was going on in the professional departments but she also knew all the people who made the hospital run. She helped me navigate both levels – the departmental level and the underground: the mailroom, photography, food services, buildings and grounds and security. When security cameras recorded a chief of service having sex with a colleague in a conference room, information about the incident went quickly through the underground to Beverly. She told me and we had a good laugh.

16

· · · · ·

Groundbreaking
Discovery
The HD Gene

My first years at Mass General were very exciting scientifically. Faculty members Rudy Tanzi, Jim Gusella and their collaborators found the gene for one form of Alzheimer's disease and Robert Brown found another gene for one form of amyotrophic lateral sclerosis (ALS).

Since 1981, I had continued to go to Venezuela yearly to get samples from patients that would bring us closer to identifying the actual Huntington's disease genetic mutation. In 1983, two years after starting the hunt for the Huntington's gene, a marker was discovered that tracked through the family with those who had the disease. That marker was *not* the gene – rather just a random piece of DNA that flowed through the HD family tree nearby the actual HD gene. This was a big milestone to reach even though the mutation itself in the gene was still unknown.

Finally, ten years after finding the marker, the project paid off. At the end of February 1993, Marcy MacDonald and Jim Gusella told Nancy and me that they had found the actual mutation in the gene for Huntington's disease! Since the discovery of the marker, it had taken what Natalie Angier, in her article that was later published on the front page of the *New York Times*, called "ten years of backbreaking work" to find the mutation. The process itself had also been extraordinary – six separate laboratories had worked so closely together that they agreed to publish their findings together in the March issue of *Cell* – authorship was credited to them as a collaborative group. This was quite an unusual practice for scientists who typically compete to be first or best to make a discovery. What a joyous day!

Now we knew that the HD gene mutation was composed of an abnormal number of repeated sequences in the DNA, which was in keeping with what other research scientists had already found to be the cause of several other neurologic diseases. Simply put, DNA is an instruction manual for our bodies. The instructions are written in three-letter words made from an alphabet of four letters: A, T, G, C. The three-letter words each encode an amino acid. In what are called 'triplet repeat disorders,' one 'word' is stuttered and repeated many times. The more repeats, the earlier the onset of the disease. For HD, it was a CAG repeat – CAG codes for the amino acid, glutamine. All people have the HD gene; in most healthy people, there are less than 30 CAG repeats. People with the actual disease have more than 36 CAG repeats.

The identification of the gene mutation allowed for many new experiments to be done. Our own lab (affectionately known for years as the 'Flying Pig' laboratory) and the labs of many others throughout the world started to look at the distribution of the mutant gene and the resulting protein (termed *huntingtin*) in the postmortem brain. In Michigan, we had collected a large number of HD postmortem brains and we brought many of them to Boston.

In particular, we had the brain of an at-risk person we'd identified in our prospective PET scan study. She had been at-risk for HD because of her family history but had no symptoms. She had been followed annually for three years when she committed suicide. A nurse, she knew how to start an IV on herself and inject a high concentration of potassium chloride, which stopped her heart immediately but preserved her brain exquisitely. Her family found her hours after her death and generously donated her brain for research. This tragedy allowed us to see the earliest changes in an at-risk human brain. It also showed inclusions (clumps of the huntingtin protein) in the nerve cells of her HD brain. Our lab used different techniques to view both the gene distribution and protein localization in this at-risk brain and in the brains of many other patients we had followed over the years.

Other research was made possible after finding the gene mutation because lab investigators could now insert the HD gene mutation as a 'transgene' in animals such as mice, fruit flies, pigs, sheep and monkeys. The so-called transgenic HD animals became ill over time just like the human disease. These animals made it possible for scientists to examine the function of the protein and design possible therapies.

The identification of the gene mutation also made possible a simple blood test that allowed people to determine whether they had inherited HD. At first, there was some enthusiasm for getting tested. However, it soon became clear by the relative few who signed up for the test that many people would rather live with ambiguity than know they would definitely develop a deadly, incurable disease sometime in the future. It was clearly a personal, difficult decision to take the test. Nancy, Ira, Jack, I and other clinicians discussed the best approach to genetic testing and our guidelines were adopted by clinicians. In addition to genetic counseling, a candidate for testing should have both a neurological and psychiatric evaluation to make sure they were not depressed or suicidal. A candidate should come to these evaluation meetings with a supportive and trusted companion. Results should be given in person, not over the phone. Finding out whether one carried the HD gene mutation opened a whole Pandora's box of problems. Who can access the information? Can you be fired from your job because you carry the gene mutation? What about healthcare and insurance? The answers to these questions were unknown. Some progress has since been made with the 2008 passage of the Genetic Information Nondiscrimination Act (GINA) and the 2019 Genetic Information Privacy Act (GIPA). Both of these acts have their problems and more work is necessary for the future.

Nancy was asked by James Watson (discoverer of DNA) to head the Ethical, Legal and Social Issues (ELSI) committee of the nascent Human Genome Project at the NIH to define guidelines for genetic testing, protection of genetic information, legality of privacy and the social implications of genetic testing. Ironically, because of the work she had done to find the gene, Nancy now had to face the difficult decision of whether she wanted to get tested. Should she do it? What would she gain by being tested? She had no children but she had wanted them. She knew too well what it was like to have the disease. Ultimately both Nancy and her sister, Alice, remained private about being tested. Diane Sawyer interviewed Nancy, Alice and Milton Wexler for *60 Minutes* discussing their thoughts about testing. Hearing Nancy talk in the interview about her decision to remain private gave permission to other at-risk persons to do the same.

Finally, the discovery of the gene mutation allowed the possibility of preimplantation diagnosis of embryos. Women who knew they were at-risk for carrying the gene mutation and elected to get pregnant by in vitro fertilization (IVF) could undergo an egg retrieval, which would be fertilized in the lab with sperm, and then any viable embryos that grew in the petri dish could be tested for the HD gene mutation. Only HD mutation-free embryos would be implanted into the woman's womb. This development made it possible for families to have children free of HD. No longer did a child have to inherit a 50 percent chance of developing HD if one of their parents carried the gene mutation.

I was overjoyed by the discovery of the HD gene mutation. Our lab worked hard on examining the location of the huntingtin protein in the brain. We worked closely with Marian DiFiglia, an outstanding Mass General neuroanatomist. It was very intense but also fun work. Jack and I ran our lab and I still had to run the large department.

In the summer, we visited Jack's father and stepmother, Nancy, in New Hampshire, often driving up for the day. We loved Bow Lake. Jack's dad rented a little trailer each year down by the water to keep windsurfers, a canoe and a motorboat. The lake was delicious but we didn't go often to Jack's family farm because it made us both sad to see how all the things that Jack's mother had taken pride in had been neglected since she'd died. The family china had been broken and the silverware lost. Staying overnight was not encouraged because all the bedrooms were filled with piles of extra clothing and boxes of knick-knacks.

We decided that the best strategy was to buy a house of our own on the lake. After more than six months, we found a really beautiful house for sale by the owner. It was a camp that had been fully winterized and modernized. The top floor was the main floor and the above-ground basement was fitted out with a washer/dryer, freezers, a workbench and plenty of room for extra beds and storage for windsurfer sails and boards. It had a beautiful screened porch and living room/dining room that looked out over the lake and two islands that were about 100 yards off shore. It faced southeast, which was not ideal for windsurfing, but that disappointment was made up for by its sandy beach and long dock. The problem was it cost too much. We waited. After six months nobody had bought it. The interest rates were nearing an all-time low and we were putting away more money. We decided to make an offer below the asking price and miraculously the sellers accepted almost immediately.

Now we had our own house. We had accumulated plenty of dishes and old furniture that we moved to the lake house and furnished it instantly, buying almost nothing except for a big hot tub that we put outside under the dining room window. It was a perfect place to spend the weekends all year round in sun, snow or rain. It was a perfect place to have lab parties. Boston was only an hour and a half away, yet it was a totally different environment with the smells of the tall white pines and the calls of loons. At night, all year long, you could sit in the hot tub and see the stars and comets.

After the discovery of the HD mutation, Jack joined up with his friend, Ira Shoulson, to start the Huntington Study Group (HSG) modeled after the Parkinson Study Group that the two had formed nine years earlier. The goal of the HSG was to form a multi-institutional coalition of HD experts who agreed to use common tools and strategies to evaluate patients and quickly enter them into clinical trials. I was appointed head of the Scientific Affairs Committee of the HSG. Over the ensuing years, the HSG conducted many clinical trials in HD and still continues over 30 years later.

I had a patient who worked for Apple, and from him I learned how computers were now able to communicate with each other at institutions or companies all over the country. He told me how the many franchises of the Domino's Pizza chain communicated all at once through a computer network. In 1993, a faculty member sent me one of her lab technicians, John Lester, who said he would like to set up the department on a computerized network and connect us to the World Wide Web, which was just starting to become more widely used. I immediately hired him. Our department was the first at the hospital to be on the web. Now all faculty and residents could easily communicate. John set up collaborative Brain Communities for people with rare neurological diseases and their families all over the world to connect with each other online. Those with rare or crippling disorders who otherwise didn't know fellow sufferers or who couldn't leave the house could now interact with others with their same afflictions. It worked beautifully for several years but eventually the hospital told us to close the communities down when some members started abusing them. To continue, it would be necessary to edit all entries and that was too expensive for us. A decade later, MySpace and Facebook came online to provide this sort of shared community.

In 1994, shortly after Sam became president of Mass General, a merger between Mass General and Brigham was announced. Sam had only been president of Mass General for a couple of years before becoming the first president of what was and still is the even larger Partners HealthCare System (now called Mass General Brigham). Of course I had to think about what the merger meant for neurology and other departments. Would all the departments be expected to merge with their counterparts? Who would lead the departments? What did the merger mean for me?

One challenge of the merger was how to deal with departments like neurology. At the Brigham, it was not a distinct department but rather a division of the medicine department. If Partners really wanted us to merge, the resulting department should truly be one with one leader at the top. I thought that it would be key to first make neurology a full-fledged department at the Brigham. Later, I could become head of a combined department. That way I could coordinate subspecialty clinics, clinical trials and basic research across the two departments. I had both the clinical and basic research expertise to be successful. I talked about it with Sam, and he asked me to write up a proposal supporting a plan in which I would be a co-chair with Marty Samuels, who was then head of the Division of Neurology at the Brigham. I wrote up a plan and showed it to Sam, who said he liked it and thought it would work. But when he took it to the leadership at the Brigham, the plan was initially rejected. Sam said it was because the five department chairs at the Brigham didn't want another person to join their inner sanctum. I thought I was the candidate most qualified to become head of a combined department since I was a clinician, scientist and teacher. Marty was not an academic researcher. He was a teacher – and an outstanding one at that. He was promoted on a special new track called the Teacher Clinician Track.

Despite this initial rejection, I worked hard for neurology to become a department at Brigham. I was still hoping that I'd be designated the overall leader with Marty acting as a local Brigham neurology vice chair reporting to me. In the end, neurology did become a full department at the Brigham and Marty and I were designated co-chairs and had to collaborate on everything.

My colleagues were surprised with the co-chair idea and commiserated with me about how I had gotten the short end of the stick in the deal. I just learned to live with it since I had no inclination to move to a new institution. Jack supported me through this, comforted me, told me he loved me and said I was doing a great job as head of the Mass General department.

As president of Partners HealthCare System, Sam played a big role in recruiting Jim Mongan as the next president of Mass General. Jim had never worked in Boston. He came by a circuitous route from San Francisco and Stanford to the Department of Health and Human Services in Washington, DC in the Carter administration and ultimately to Kansas, where he had been executive director of the Truman Medical Center in Kansas City and dean of the University of Missouri–Kansas City School of Medicine.

What a great guy! Jim was an unassuming, oh-gosh kind of guy who had a keen sense of humor that often led to side-splitting laughter. Deals were made above the board and as public knowledge. Strategic plans were laid out to the leadership and the rest of us were invited to become collaborative partners in figuring out how to reach a common goal. He listened carefully, but more importantly, he had the great skill of distilling the essence of a long discussion or contentious argument into three or four key issues. If an issue was cloaked in secrecy or mired in politics, he exposed it, washed it off and displayed it cleanly to all. He was fair to all the services, regardless of whether they made any revenue for the hospital. He was a wonderful leader.

Every year, we recruited a new set of residents. The applicants were brilliant, dedicated, fun and enthusiastic. Each November, we had an intense recruitment effort interviewing as many as 50 applicants for 6 slots. We interviewed candidates from US medical schools but also from Europe, the Middle East and India. The applicants were part of a Neurology Match. Each applicant submitted a ranked list of their highest program choices to the Match. The institutions also submitted their ranked list of applicants. We usually matched many of our favorite choices. In 1994, after Mass General and the Brigham merged as Partners, we joined our previously separate residency programs into a single large program with 18 residents each year. Our combined program was very popular, and we were lucky to continue to recruit great people from diverse scientific and personal backgrounds.

The residents had an intense training schedule. Every third night, three first-year residents stayed in the hospital and so did a third-year resident. On any given night, there were at least four neurology residents at the hospital. By being there all night, the residents helped each other out, shared the cases and learned more by working together than they would have alone. The residents bonded together, and many became friends for the rest of their lives. Over the course of their three-year training, our faculty also got to know the residents very well. We could observe their strengths and weaknesses. In a way, they were our 'farm' team from which we could scout future junior faculty.

One of our residents, Alice Flaherty, had obtained her PhD with our friend, the famous neuroanatomist Ann Graybiel at MIT. Ann had made important discoveries about the striatum, the largest nucleus within the basal ganglia. When we were in Michigan, Jack and I had spent time with her discussing the circuitry of the basal ganglia on our trips to Boston. Alice had done beautiful neuroscience work in Ann's lab, and I hoped I could recruit her to work in my laboratory as a fellow after she finished her residency. She decided, however, not to pursue lab work but rather to do a movement disorders fellowship. Whenever we worked together in the outpatient clinic, she was fun to talk to about the best ways to support patients through the difficult times in their illness. She and her husband had both spent time at the University of Michigan, so we had that in common also. Alice became a talented clinician, and when her fellowship was over, I asked her to join the faculty. She accepted and soon had an office near mine and Beverly's. I liked to see patients with her because she had a fund of interesting information about nervous system disease.

Three of my former Michigan MD/PhD students were accepted into the Mass General neurology residency program. Each had studied different glutamate receptors in the rat and human brain. Jang-Ho Cha worked on AMPA receptors, Claudia Testa on metabotropic glutamate receptors and Sharin Sakarai on NMDA receptors. I knew how dedicated and motivated they were in the lab and was sure they would be great residents. Jang-Ho Cha decided to work in our laboratory after his residency and he carried out the first neurotransmitter receptor evaluations of HD transgenic mice. A good friend in London, HD gene hunter and geneticist Gill Bates, had put a piece of the human HD gene into a mouse. Every cell in the mouse body shared the piece. The

267

animals were okay at birth but gradually lost coordination, strength and weight and eventually died in about 14 weeks. The first transgenic animal model of HD! Jang-Ho was the first to examine neurotransmitter receptors in this model and found changes in the transgenic mice that suggested nerve cells lost their neurotransmitter properties long before the nerve cells died. Jang-Ho went on to form his own lab, which he ran for about a decade, but ultimately decided he could do as much or more for diseases like HD by working in the pharmaceutical industry.

A year or two after Jang-Ho's studies, Ai Yamamoto, a graduate student with Rene Hen at Columbia University, made a transgenic mouse whose HD transgene could be turned on or off in the living animal. When the gene was turned on, the animals got sick after about three months and eventually died. If the gene was turned off, even when the animals were sick, the animals would get better! This was the first time a neurodegenerative disorder had been shown to be reversible – a game-changer – indicating that, in the future, treatments could theoretically make a person *better, not just keep them from getting worse*. The notion that early in the neurodegenerative disease the cells are sick but not dead and can be potentially rescued by therapies brings hope for managing these diseases in the future.

Nancy and I also recruited people to Venezuela to help with the projects. We talked frequently on the phone and saw each other at meetings. We found we had similar intuitions about who would be best for the project. Students, residents and fellows were great participants. Over the years, more than 10 of my trainees took part in the Venezuela project and all went into neurology (Figures 16.1 and 16.2). Furthermore, most went into careers focusing on HD and other neurodegenerative disorders. They were energetic and eager to learn everything possible. Being able to teach and influence the trainees made the work and research fun. Several basic scientists also joined the Venezuela project, including Leslie

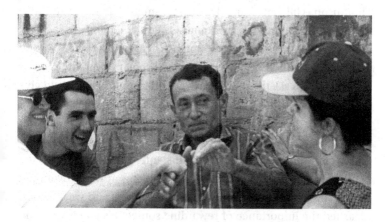

Figure 16.1 Merit Cudkowicz, Michael Grecius, a Venezuelan with HD and Diana Rosas – three Mass General neurology residents who came to Venezuela.

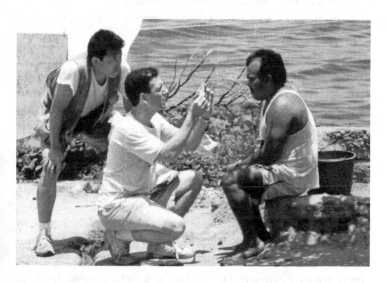

Figure 16.2 Residents Jang-Ho Cha and Hal Blumenfeld examining a Venezuelan man.

Thompson, Gill Bates and David Housman. I made many new friends during these yearly sojourns. Leslie Thompson, a basic scientist who is bilingual in Spanish, came down for several years. She was a very poised and good-looking woman. One of her jobs was to ask the men to give sperm samples. She would give them sexy magazines to aid in getting the sperm samples in a back room. Often the men would prefer that she go into the room with them and try to pull her in. She would then say: "Jack . . . ? Jack . . . ? Please come and help." Jack would instantly appear to redirect the man. Working on the project was like being at adult overnight camp. You learned everyone's foibles, strengths and weaknesses. I learned the importance of rewarding someone's good work and the value of remaining patient with those who irritated me.

In Boston, as chair of neurology, one critical issue I had to address was the recruitment and promotion of women faculty. In Michigan, I hadn't been involved in appointments and promotions and my mentors had always been supportive of me. At Mass General, I spoke to each of the women faculty and found that there were several who appeared ready for promotion. Peculiarly, though, the women never asked for anything for themselves. The male faculty had no reluctance to ask for resources, space and a salary increase. On the other hand, several of the women faculty worked for male neurologists in private practice seeing their Medicaid and nonpaying patients. The women's salaries were pathetic. I tried to emphasize how they had been manipulated by their so-called colleagues and persuade them to insist on fair pay or else leave these private practitioners.

I learned how women were essentially overlooked. Nobody was there to praise their work. None of the powerful men knew them. The guys all played golf or tennis together or went to Boston area sports events. Women just weren't on their radar screens. Harvard Medical School promotions all had to be approved first by a departmental executive committee made up of the chiefs of service at the hospitals. Unless her chief stuck up for the woman candidate, the promotion would be questioned and fail. Many times I saw this strategy played out. A typical way of sinking a promotion was to question the candidate's value. "Yes. So-and-So published these three papers but did she really improve our understanding of a disease and can others repeat it?" So much for that applicant. If her chief didn't speak up to counter this subjective evaluation and emphatically champion the candidate, the promotion would fail.

If a woman candidate survived the chiefs of service, the next obstacle was the Harvard Medical School Promotions Committee, which consisted of about 40 HMS faculty from various basic and clinical departments. Each candidate was discussed and the promotion voted on. Again, women suffered unless their chief spoke up, answering questions from other faculty and explaining any challenges to the candidate's promotion. I spoke up often. "Oh, she's positively brilliant; she has discovered new fundamental principles," I might say. Or, "I know she has a lot of important experiments in the pipeline." Over my 21 years as chief, I was able to promote women to each academic level until 30–35 percent of assistant, associate and professor levels were filled by women. When I started at Mass General, the numbers were 35 percent, 10 percent and 0 percent, respectively, for each level.

17

. . . . .

Scud Missiles

I learned quickly when I came to Boston that running a department means you spend most of your time taking care of the fallout from the few troublemakers and much less time on the really precious and productive team players. Ray was a particularly difficult faculty member. He had had a big laboratory in former years and had made a reputation in the area of pain research. By the time I came, he still occupied a large laboratory; however, he had lost his grants. He used funding from gifts and drug companies to run his lab. He also ran an active pain service at the local physical rehabilitation hospital. He played a significant role in the pain service at Mass General. People came to see me complaining about how he was disrupting all the interactive programs of the service, how he used his fellows as his lackeys at the hospital and how nobody could ever find him to discuss his assigned patients.

He had made an impression years before when during an NIH site visit for his program project grant on pain mechanisms, he had made an advance on one of the women site visitors during the laboratory tours and was reported to the head of the department and head of the site visit team. It was hard to believe that such an inappropriate person could exist at Mass General but it was apparently true.

I got complaints from faculty colleagues and his postdoctoral fellows that he was impossible to trust or to deal with. His fellows seemed to hate him as he used them and never made an effort to enhance their careers, only his own. I counseled him several times about how it was in his best interest to gain the trust of his colleagues and his fellows. I impressed upon him how vital it is to one's career to have trainees that respect him and laud him rather than despise and distrust him. He nodded and implied that he understood and explained how all of this had nothing to do with him but rather it was the fault of the others.

I decided I had to take his laboratory away as he had no federal or foundation funding. This didn't seem to faze him. When I later encouraged him to leave the institution, he didn't complain but rather went off to another institution in town to join a private practice.

It was only years later that I read in the newspapers that he was being reprimanded and suspended by the Massachusetts Board of Medical Registration for secretly taping his secretary in compromising situations.

People like Ray would require me to meet for hours with many faculty, fellows and secretaries and take me away from my laboratory work – since that time was most flexible. I call these incidents 'Scud missiles' because they come in completely unexpectedly and destroy my schedule.

Other situations involve faculty who have done nothing wrong but who are influenced by the rules and regulations set for the faculty. The hospital and medical school sometimes didn't think carefully about certain organizational issues. I was at Chief's Council (all department heads at Mass General) one morning when Gerald Austen, chair of the Council, brought out a letter. Austen said the letter was from some guy named John Penney who was pointing out that the Nominating Committee of the Mass General Physician's Organization often put its own members on the ballot. The letter said members who were on the nominating committee should not be running for any current office. I spoke up to tell the Council that John Penney was my husband, Jack, and that he was right in his comments. Jack's suggestions to prevent such conflicts of interest in this respect were adopted.

Sometimes the conflicts of interest are more obvious. Most people go into science because they find it rewarding to think up a problem or hypothesis (or to address somebody else's hypothesis or problem), devise an experiment to test the hypothesis and then come up with a definitive result. They are less driven by the desire to make money. University positions pay low salaries compared to what one could earn in the private sector. They are rewarded by fame and academic stature. But these drives are relative.

Yet scientists are human beings and even they like to 'luck out' and make millions. After all, they may think they have 'sacrificed' their careers to help better mankind and deserve some reward. Why can't they hold equity in a company that they helped found and be paid by the company to conduct their academic or clinical research? Here's why: Even if somebody is the smartest, most equitable and humble person, human nature is to 'want' the experiment to turn out a certain way – maybe the result will make millions of dollars. Ditto for a scientist who designs a new drug or device to cure a disease (or other problem) – a conflict of interest means that holding equity in the company that makes the drug or device will inevitably affect an investigator's clinical trials to test its efficacy. Clinical trials can be influenced even when only part of a multisite program is affected.

Conflict of interest issues are also rife in consulting. Suppose a company is willing to pay a member of its scientific advisory board $25,000 a year but the university limits consulting fees to $10,000 a year. Most people who serve on a scientific advisory board would support an increase in the limits of the payments if such a change was proposed.

These issues became especially relevant at Mass General in 1998. Joe Martin had recently become dean of the medical school and a committee of Harvard Medical School professors was assembled to reconsider the guidelines for conflict of interest. Quite a buzz developed at the meetings attended by chiefs of service.

Finally, when formal presentations on the proposed new financial guidelines were presented, it soon became obvious something more was afoot than a simple guideline reevaluation. I was one of two people who spoke against any loosening of the existing stringent guidelines. At first, I was perplexed by the number of crossed arms, scowling faces and turned-away torsos that greeted any criticism of the potential guideline changes. Only when I returned to my office did I realize that almost everybody on the committee to reevaluate the guidelines stood to gain personally by the proposed changes. At the next meeting in which the guidelines were discussed, I and one other faculty member, again, spoke against the guideline changes and, again, the body language in the room changed.

I decided to speak up about this uneasiness. I said I found it disturbing that people in the room had provided such intense support for the changes particularly since they themselves might benefit by the changes. Immediately, people protested that there was absolutely *no way* they would let a potential monetary gain influence their evaluation of the issues. Fortunately, the dean listened carefully to all the input and decided to table the issue and keep the rules as they were for the near future. It was clear, however, that I had lost a few brownie points with several of the more aggressive chiefs of service.

275

Issues around conflicts of interest continue to play a big role in academic medicine, particularly in the past two decades, during which many scientists in universities have received funding from industry and have, in fact, started small biotechnology companies in which they have equity. A small number of people have reaped very large rewards, and just like the lottery, many scientists secretly (or not so secretly) wish that they could strike it rich also.

Other sources of trouble arose from the fact that hospitals competed for people and resources. Leaders at one hospital might try to take over programs at another hospital. One such incident happened to me with the president of Dana Farber. He had been chair of pediatrics at Children's Hospital and then became president of the Dana Farber Cancer Institute. He asked to meet with me and the Mass General heads of neurosurgery and the Cancer Center because Dana Farber wanted to put in a large grant to the National Cancer Institute to support brain tumor research. In particular, the Dana Farber president wanted to have a certain young medical oncologist at the Dana Farber lead the project and run brain tumor research across the Harvard hospitals. This particular candidate had no training in neuro-oncology and had only recently been promoted to assistant professor. I told the Dana Farber president that I could not support his suggested candidate because this man had a poor reputation for collaboration. Furthermore, a guy in *my* department, who ran our brain tumor clinical and basic research, was an associate professor and a trained neuro-oncologist with grants. He would be a more appropriate leader. Looking straight at me, the Dana Farber president said that he had already made up his mind and that it was up to me to *make* my people like this young man. I said I had no intention of making any of my faculty put up with let alone *like* anybody. I said that the young oncologist had not made any friends at Mass General and that spoke for itself.

At this point the other two left the room for reasons I forget now. When I was alone with him, the Dana Farber president insisted that I really had to appoint his candidate and that if I did not he threatened to make me regret it and to switch his allegiances to the neurologists at the Beth Israel Hospital. This was the final blow! Who the hell did he think he was? The Beth Israel Hospital was then in a competitive hospital network to that of the Mass General, Brigham and the Dana Farber. I told him he could do as he wished but that I wasn't going to go against my principles.

We ended our conversation. The first thing I did was call up Sam Thier, the head of Partners HealthCare. I told him of this ridiculous behavior. I knew that I would have no influence on the Dana Farber president but Sam was fair and powerful. The next day, Sam called me to say that he had taken care of the bully and I had nothing to worry about.

Of course, I knew before I came Harvard can be a brutal place. Faculty lives were consumed and regurgitated with little concern for the consequences. Rivalry between the hospitals was intense. One such instance involved a junior faculty member who was used as a pawn by the hospital leadership to access resources unethically. I learned all the gory details after the damage had already been done because I was on a committee to investigate. Here's how the duplicitous behind-the-scenes dealings played out.

The Brigham and the Dana Farber Cancer Institute were in desperate need of a new linear accelerator for state-of-the-art cancer treatment. The Commonwealth of Massachusetts however, regulates the number of these expensive and highly specialized devices and had already distributed so-called certificates of need (CONs) for them within the state. At about the same time, the position of head of the Radiation Oncology Division became open at the Brigham and a search for a new director of the division had been approved by Harvard Medical School. Two members of the search committee were the head of radiation oncology at the Beth Israel Hospital and the chief medical officer at the Brigham.

The presidents of the Brigham and Dana Farber Cancer Institute were keen on acquiring a CON for a new linear accelerator and it turned out that the Beth Israel had two CONs – one for an older device that was now essentially obsolete and another for one that had recently been purchased. Beth Israel was approached about selling their outdated device along with its CON to the Brigham and Dana Farber Cancer Institute. Once purchased, the Brigham and Dana Farber Cancer Institute could ditch the old device and buy a new one because they could still use the CON of the older device.

While all this was going on, the search committee was busy screening potential candidates for the vacant position as head of Brigham Radiation Oncology. As I've said, the holder of the equivalent role at Beth Israel was on the search committee, but he also wanted the job himself, which represented a conflict of interest. He'd submitted an application regardless, and the presidents of the Brigham and the Dana Farber Cancer Institute along with the chief medical officer of the Brigham asked him not to say anything about wanting the job and to withdraw his application for fear that Beth Israel may withdraw their offer to sell their old device and CON. In return for his silence, they told him they would appoint him as head of the Brigham Radiation Oncology once the deal for the CON had gone through. They told him to ignore what the search committee was doing, as they would bypass the search committee's recommendation and ensure he got the role.

Once the Beth Israel head of radiation oncology withdrew his candidacy, the search committee began to earnestly look at other candidates. After reviewing a broad group, they settled on one leading candidate who was a young assistant professor at Beth Israel Hospital who was a protégé of the head of radiation oncology. Although she was young, she was an MD–PhD and had proved herself to be a very viable candidate with excellent scholarship and leadership skills. They decided she was the top candidate for the job.

In considering the job, she called her mentor the head of radiation oncology at the Beth Israel Hospital on multiple occasions to ask advice about the job. Was this the right move at this time in her career? Would he still help her as she fashioned a new division? At no point did he say that he, in fact, wanted the job or relay the fact that the leadership had offered him the job on the side. The chief medical officer at the Brigham who was on the search committee also made no effort to inform the committee that the head of radiation oncology at the Beth Israel was the preferred candidate of the hospital. In fact, he met with the young woman and discussed the position and its accompanying responsibilities with her.

As the search committee was winding up its activities, the head of radiation oncology at Beth Israel began to doubt the sincerity of the leadership at the Brigham and Dana Farber. He bumped into the president of the Dana Farber at a cocktail party and he was reassured that he was still their candidate. He told them that the search committee had chosen his younger colleague as the candidate. Again he was reassured but sworn to secrecy because of the CON.

The search committee announced their choice of the young woman, and it was announced at the annual meeting of the Radiation Oncology Society. It was the talk of the meeting; all her colleagues congratulated her on her new position. At this point the deal with the Beth Israel Hospital for the CON was done and the CON was transferred. Upon sealing the deal, the presidents of the Brigham and Dana Farber called the head of radiation oncology at Beth Israel and offered him the position of head of the Division at the Brigham. He accepted immediately. He questioned what would happen to his young colleague and mentee and was told that unfortunately she had to live with the decision. What about the search committee and its deliberations? He was told that the hospital position was not at the discretion of the medical school and was a hospital administrative position. The search committee was irrelevant. The hospital could appoint whoever they wanted.

The woman was contacted by the chief medical officer at the Brigham. He told her that she no longer had the appointment because the hospital had decided to appoint her boss at the Beth Israel Hospital to the position. She was shocked. Her boss was on the search committee and had never mentioned the decision of the Brigham administration. Why hadn't he been up-front with the search committee and informed them that their deliberations were pointless? He backpedaled and hemmed and hawed. She went to the dean of Harvard Medical School who was then Joe Martin, and also my predecessor in neurology at Mass General. He was taken aback by the developments. The young woman soon became the detritus of the academic process when she had to tell her colleagues (and everyone in the field for that matter) that she didn't actually get the position. She felt abandoned and humiliated. What would she do? Stay in her same position? What would happen if her mentor played a role in her upcoming promotion to associate professor? She felt powerless.

Joe contacted the presidents of the hospitals and expressed his concern about their conduct. He was told that they regretted the young woman's humiliation but reinforced their right to appoint the new head of radiation oncology as they pleased. The young woman asked Joe for a formal investigation of the integrity of the presidents of the Brigham and Dana Farber, the Brigham chief medical officer and the new Brigham head of radiation oncology. How could they allow the search committee to proceed in its deliberations knowing they had a preferred candidate who had formally withdrawn from candidacy? How could the chief medical officer meet with her as a candidate knowing she would not get the job? How could they be so callous as to let a young faculty member be humiliated in front of all her professional colleagues? How could her former mentor advise her about the pros and cons of the new position and never mention the fact that he was secretly the preferred candidate?

That was when Joe asked me to join a committee to look into the allegations of the young woman. And after an in-depth deliberation, we advised him as dean to strongly reprimand the leadership of the Brigham and Dana Farber and to put the new head of radiation oncology at the Brigham on probation and remove him from any role in subsequent deliberations for the promotion of the young woman.

The recommendations were implemented but unfortunately the water was under the bridge and the real casualty of all the activities was the young woman who was caught in the arrogance of the older male leaders of the hospitals and the ruthlessness of the politics. I learned that senior leaders of the medical community were willing to sacrifice junior faculty to get the desired institutional results. From then on, when navigating my department through institutional mazes, I kept this lesson in mind.

Scud missiles took on various forms. Not only did they take me away from my research and students but they were stressful. I would awake every night around 3 a.m. and worry about all the politics and meetings I had ahead. I learned to use this nighttime wakefulness to solve some of my issues emotionally. I made decisions. I also practiced lectures and presentations in the middle of the night. I figured I added an hour or two of work each night but my work was never done. There was always more to take care of and accomplish.

Particularly painful were times when a faculty member was accused of scientific misconduct or plagiarism. I got an email from one of my faculty. She had just come back from a gene therapy meeting where she was accused of plagiarism. A postdoctoral fellow in her laboratory gave a presentation and one of the slides (given to him by another fellow in her lab) looked virtually identical to a figure already published by a woman in the audience. The woman contacted the president of the Society of Gene Therapy and claimed that her data had been plagiarized. My faculty member immediately called the fellow who said that the data was his and that it was just a coincidence that the data looked so much like that published by the accuser. In fact, he said, his data were simply confirmatory of the woman's data. I was told the fellow had looked through his desk and lab bench and been unable to locate the experiment in question. The president of the society was asking for an investigation. We notified the director of research affairs at Mass General. The fellow's notebooks, lab data and computer were possessed and he was barred from the lab until the investigation was completed.

I was shocked by the whole affair. The fellow had been one of our residents and had always been an outstanding doctor and team player. He had been successful in obtaining a competitive research training grant from the National Institutes of Health. I just couldn't believe that he would ever plagiarize. There was no apparent motivation, plus he had always seemed like the most solid of characters. He had his grant, a child on the way and he was about to take the neurology boards.

The original slide presented at the meeting was given to me along with a copy of the article from which the data were allegedly copied. I locked it in my office. The Mass General director of research affairs said that we should ask the fellow to replicate the data if he could not find the original gel and that he should do so under the supervision of a faculty member that had expertise in the experimental approach. Unfortunately, after several months the data still could not be replicated. At this point, however, the Mass

General decided to report the case to Harvard Medical School for adjudication.

The medical school formed a review committee to begin deliberations. Several faculty members reviewed the data and met with the fellow to see if they could repeat the data. They could not. I met with the fellow and asked him about the proceedings and whether he had an explanation for the whole affair. He denied having done anything wrong and expressed the fact that he was perplexed by the whole proceedings. He emphasized that he had no motivation to plagiarize. He didn't actually publish the data and it certainly wasn't likely to move him ahead scientifically. He admitted that he had included the figure in question in a grant application to the National Institutes of Health.

The suspicion was that a digital copy of the figure had been made and then altered in something like Adobe Photoshop. A report was sent to the Office of Scientific Integrity at the National Institutes of Health.

It took four months for the NIH Office of Scientific Integrity to interview people and analyze the data. They got an expert to get the fellow's old files off his computer and compare them with digital copies of the figure from the journal. They provided specific evidence that the figure had indeed been copied and then doctored up in Photoshop. We confronted the fellow and it was only then he admitted that he had copied the figure. He said he was not able to spend enough time on his experiments with his new baby and the neurology board exams coming up. He was scared that he wouldn't get his first independent research project and that his career would be compromised. As a result of all this he was banned from eligibility for NIH grants for five years. He had to resign from HMS and the Mass General and went into private practice neurology.

I was personally hurt by his feeling that only plagiarism would rescue him from failure because I had always tried to emphasize to my junior faculty that I would try to find them interim funding if they ever had a funding gap. Considering him a personal friend, I had hoped that if he was insecure about his career he would come to me for help and advice.

Early in the whole process I had met with Dean Joe Martin and told him about the case and about my suspicions of his innocence. Joe's primary point to me was, "you're often surprised by these cases where the person is so seemingly the innocent type." What a tragedy for a talented young clinician scientist. He had so much promise to be a success in his career and under stress he committed an egregious error.

18

• • • • •

Designing a New Research Center

Our laboratories were on the main Mass General campus next to the hospital. Other neurology labs were in the Charlestown Navy Yard. Most scientists worked in laboratories whose doors could be closed and separated from other labs. Scientists could occupy side-by-side laboratories and never get to know their neighbors. Jack and I began to wonder whether we could put all the neurology laboratories working on neurodegenerative disorders in one space where they could all collaborate together. Neurodegenerative disorders had common features such as intracellular protein inclusions, genetic factors, aging, metabolic stress and progressive loss of specific subpopulations of nerve cells. In Alzheimer's disease, the hippocampus and cerebral cortex are damaged; in Parkinson's disease, the problem is with the dopamine cells of the brainstem; in Huntington's disease, it's the striatal and cortical neurons; and in amyotrophic lateral sclerosis (ALS), the motor cells of the cerebral cortex and spinal cord are damaged. Factors causing one disease might have implications for the other diseases as well. If we could all work side by side, we might together come up with potential therapies sooner. Therapies working in one neurodegenerative disease might work in the others too. The idea was to put the labs of collaborative investigators in contiguous laboratories with no walls or doors between them. This design was new and unusual. Everyone would have to interact. Jack and I figured the only way to pull this off was to find new space that we could occupy.

We hoped that the new center would be designed to accelerate the development of new therapies. Perhaps we could speed up the process by addressing the barriers that existed in drug development. The 'Valley of Death' – the long gap in time between when a basic science discovery is made and when a company decides to license the intellectual property to develop a clinical application – was a major issue facing drug development. Jack and I knew that most new drugs came from fundamental basic science observations made by academics who were not inclined to pursue the actual development of a drug. Furthermore, academic faculty members were generally poor at patenting their lab discoveries. Another complication in drug development was that once academic research data is published, it is in the public domain and a company can't patent it and make a profit. A drug company is not inclined to take on a project that isn't patented. If, however, the drug company could license an academic lab's patents, they might later decide to develop a drug based on the patent's approach.

Could we speed up the drug discovery process by doing drug discovery directly in the center to narrow the time gap – the Valley of Death – between observation and manufacturing? Instead of waiting for a company to pick up a technique or idea, we could look for drugs right in the center's labs and then shop the idea around to drug companies. We would encourage our lab people to patent their observations; to support those efforts, I recruited a member of the Intellectual Property Office to come and speak with our investigators on a regular basis. We planned to create a special robotic drug screening laboratory whose sole goal would be to develop assays to screen thousands of compounds for new drugs right in our academic laboratories. The head of the special robotic screening lab would make it their job to scope out any exciting new possibilities by wandering around the labs talking to lab heads, postdocs and technicians. Anything we found could then be patented and ultimately developed into a drug in collaboration with a pharmaceutical company who licensed our patents. In the past, companies came to new drugs in a somewhat haphazard way. Our approach would allow a bridge over the Valley of Death that would shorten the drug discovery process. This direct and coordinated approach could take years off the development of effective therapies.

Who should be part of the center? I realized that certain investigators were naturally insular and reluctant to open up their labs and minds to collaborations. Some faculty were in constant competition with people inside and outside the institution. Others, however, were very open to working with colleagues and discussing their hypotheses about how things might work. I wanted to make sure that people got the most out of being in a vibrant, exciting, positive environment. I had always worked harder when the research was fun and collaborative. Creating an environment where people *wanted* to go to work each day and be with their friends and collaborators was ideal.

Besides Jack and I, logical occupants of the new center were Rudy Tanzi and Robert Brown who were working on Alzheimer's and the genetics of aging and ALS and neuromuscular disease, respectively. They were definitely fun and collaborative. Brad Hyman and Marian DiFiglia working on Alzheimer's and Parkinson's and Huntington's diseases would round out the senior faculty of the center. Each of these investigators now occupied labs in different buildings. If they moved to our new research center, they would constitute the core of the center's senior faculty. Plenty of room for junior investigators was also available. Furthermore, the senior investigators' freed-up space in other buildings would be available for faculty in other departments.

Fortunately, I was put on several committees at Mass General and one of them – the Space Committee – was examining the potential for acquiring additional research space. All the departmental requests for space were added up and adjusted for either 5 percent, 10 percent or 15 percent growth rate each year. This enormous appetite for space came to about a million square feet of new space in the next five years. Where was it going to come from? I learned what real estate was ready for renovation and what parcels of land were potential for new buildings. The first potential new building the Mass General would have available was in the Charlestown Navy Yard near the already existing enormous Mass General research building, which was Building 149, where about 750,000 square feet was distributed over 10 floors. The new building, Building 114, was a burnt-out shell, but if renovated, it would be about 70,000 square feet of lab space and additional space for conference rooms. Lifeboats for the Navy had been produced in this building – a very fitting metaphor for what I wanted to propose as the building's new purpose.

I learned that no specific request for Building 114 had been submitted. I reasoned that this new space might be perfect for the center idea that Jack and I had envisioned. How could I design the center so other departments would also get some benefit from neurology occupying the new building? From my work on the Space Committee, I knew who needed space and where it might be best for them. I went to each department chair to see if we could negotiate a space swap and what they would want in return. I was able to propose a series of moves that would make everybody happy.

I wrote a proposal to set up a new center (Figure 18.1). The center's mission was to accelerate the search for cures for neurodegenerative disease. I summarized our whole plan to have open interactive labs along with a robotic drug screening lab and colonies of transgenic animals. The goal was to get the Mass General key researchers working on neurodegenerative diseases and put them into the new open lab building. Only those researchers who I thought were welcoming, collaborative and enthusiastic would be included. Collaborations between labs would be fostered by setting up fellowships for individuals who would drive the projects. New assays for high-throughput drug

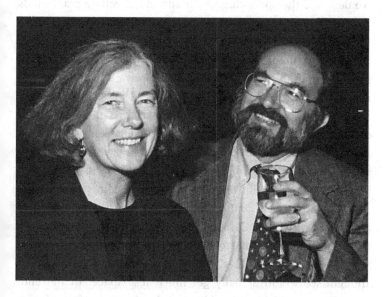

Figure 18.1 Me and Jack celebrating the plans for the new research center. Courtesy of the Hereditary Disease Foundation.

screening would be applied as soon as possible to capitalize on the finding. As soon as compounds were identified, the plan would be to partner with industry to develop them.

A wealthy man with Huntington's disease in his family approached me about trying to speed up the hunt for a cure for the disease. With his help, we set up a committee of me, Nancy and several accomplished scientists to advise him about supporting research projects at several institutions to accelerate the discovery of a therapy. We became friends and I told him about my plans for a center that would really help get to a cure more quickly. He said he would donate $2 million to get the center up and running. This was the ticket! I detailed a whole plan with various lab moves. I justified our need for the space not only because of the compelling rationale for the center but because we deserved the space due to our success at getting grant funds and because of the philanthropic funds we had been given. I asked for the entire building!

The space management people were impressed and intrigued by our proposal. No one else had come forward with any sort of coherent program for the building. We had made our case very convincingly. Multiple meetings took place over the next several months with the Space Committee, department chairs and president of Mass General. Finally, I had to present my case to the Board of Trustees of Mass General because the institution would have to commit financially to the building. Each of the meetings went well, and at each step we were encouraged to continue. When the decision was finally made, however, we were told that we could only have two-thirds of the building because of all the other space requests. Wonderful! I had thought we would actually get much less space. In the end, neurology would get an additional 9,000 square feet of new research space. It allowed me to recruit several new young investigators.

It was January 1999 when all the moves came together and a decision was to be made. Jack had to listen to me recite all the politics. He was excited with the possibilities. He had wanted our lab to be closer to the other labs working on neurodegenerative diseases. Even though this was in the Navy Yard and away from the hospital, it was worth it. By then, we were living on Beacon Hill, a short walk from Mass General and he could always get back and forth from the hospital.

On January 23, a memorial service for E. P. Richardson, the renowned Mass General neuropathologist, was held in the Unitarian Church on Marlborough Street. Jack and Ellen left right after the service to go to Aspen, Colorado for the Winter Brain Research Conference. The meetings were held from 7:30 to 9:30 a.m., 4:30 to 6:30 p.m. and 7:30 to 9:30 p.m. During the day everyone went skiing. Ellen could go because she was still on winter session for the month. Jessie was away at college. I wasn't going because there were several important meetings about the building that I had to attend.

The memorial service was beautiful. Music and eulogies by Richardson's friends and family. As we left the service, Jack kissed me goodbye. I told him to have a good time and that I loved him. I stayed for a reception and then walked home through the Public Garden covered in snow, alone.

On Wednesday, I called Jack and told him that the meetings had gone well and that our plan for the center in Charlestown had been approved. He said, "Wow! That's great!" – a lengthy statement for Jack. Jack said that the conference was very informative and the skiing was wonderful. He told me that he'd see me late Saturday and I told him I loved him and to have a safe trip (Figure 18.2).

Friday, a bunch of us from the office went out to dinner in the North End. We all got a bit drunk but we had fun. The next morning I was up early. I had breakfast and then went to get

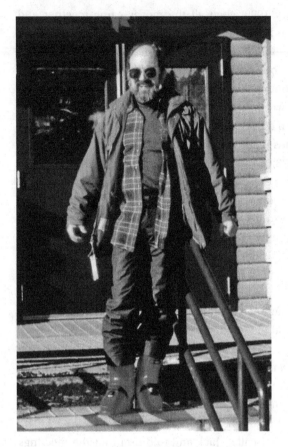

Figure 18.2 Jack in Aspen on day before death.

my hair cut. I went out for an hour-long walk along the esplanade. I was so excited about the building, and I was so glad Jack and Ellen were coming home. The Super Bowl was Sunday. In the afternoon, I worked while watching basketball. At five, I put in a potato to bake. At six, I poured myself a Jack Daniel's on ice. I put on a chop and some vegetables. After dinner, I poured myself another Jack Daniel's. At eleven, I went to bed.

At 1 a.m., I heard the buzzer at the front door and then Jack and Ellen came in and turned on the hall light. I heard Jack carry the two large suitcases up the three floors to our bedroom. Jack died that evening, an hour after getting home.

19

• • • • •

Jack's Memorial Service

After Jack's death at the end of January, it took time for me to get back into any routine at work. I was grieving and in a deep depression and trying my best to function. Beverly was a miracle. She took care of many aspects of the department with minimal input from me. Walter Koroshetz, Jane Holtz, Sherri O'Grady and Rita Zollo (Jack's secretary) all pitched in. Beverly also came to my apartment every week to go through my personal mail and help me pay my bills. Gradually, I became better able to care for myself. By March, I was spending most days in the hospital. I even went to Ann Arbor to give a lecture. Jessie was there, enrolled as a student at the University of Michigan, and I was glad to see her. Being in Ann Arbor again was painful because it reminded me more of all the good (and bad) times we had had there.

Alice Flaherty, my young colleague and trainee who helped save me with the night watch, asked me if I had gone back to my psychiatrist. I confessed to her that I never had one. She was floored. I had lied when I told her several years earlier that I had gotten help when I was really depressed. I had wanted to persuade her to see a psychiatrist during a time when she had been in such a bad way. I said it was only a partial lie since Nancy had helped me get through so many difficult times. Alice promptly made appointments for me to see two psychiatrists (pick the one you like best). She dragged me to both appointments. I settled on a psychiatrist who started me on antidepressants, and they helped but my life was still unraveling. I was going out with friends almost every night, and I drank once I got home. I wasn't on call for patient care for this first year after Jack was gone. I was in pain. It's the best word for it. I felt as if all the skin on my body was ripped off and what was left was oozing blood and pus. I never had anything to say to my psychiatrist and she just sat there until I thought up something. She told me to stop drinking and I told her I would and then kept drinking. In fact, going to see her got me thinking of alcohol and I stopped on the way home at a convenient liquor store. Alcohol eased my anger and pain.

I was going to work every day and, surprisingly, getting all my administrative work done. Patient care was always important to me and I still had pride in my clinical abilities. I continued to see outpatients one afternoon a week and I always got back to them if they called or left messages. The constant demands of the hospital were a welcome distraction. I really didn't recognize that I had a problem with alcohol. I wasn't one of those people who had a drink in the morning. I never drank before or at work or when I was on call. Throughout my career, I was never impaired while taking care of or being responsible for patients and this terrible time in my personal life was not an exception. Most of the time, though, I was not on call. The Mass General Movement Disorders group had many members and we rotated night call among us. After 6 p.m., all patient calls went to the on call attending.

There was a lot to do planning the new building – meeting with the architects and construction crews. I was awarded my own construction helmet. The building was going to be wonderful. It was on the Mystic River with full views of Boston Harbor. I had also agreed before Jack's death to give several talks at other institutions. I thought about canceling but people told me, "Oh no, that's all the more reason to come."

That said, my daughters would call and could tell if I had been drinking from my slurred speech. I would forget what they told me and I'd ask them the same questions over and over again. Ellen essentially called every night. She was terribly afraid that I would die too. Jessie was also anxious but handled it by avoiding me and the whole situation.

Both of them were managing at school despite everything. Jessie had inherited Jack's photographic memory and found most courses interesting and relatively easy. She was a botany and creative writing major and worked on her honors college thesis in her final semester. She received several prizes for her work. My daughters never talked to me about Jack. In mid May, I went to Jessie's graduation with my parents, Jack's dad and Ellen. The night before graduation, we all went to dinner and I got very tipsy. My parents mentioned nothing, but Jack's dad made a joke about my drinking that I just blew off. Graduation was in the football stadium and we could barely see Jessie, but there was another event for members of the Residential College which was smaller and more intimate. Jack, Sr. was sitting down the row from me with my parents and Ellen in between. Suddenly, Jack began to cry and sob. Nobody comforted him. I had to stand up and push my way down the aisle to give him a hug. Later, my father mentioned how pitiful it was to have a grown man cry because his oldest son couldn't see his oldest daughter graduate. I could have choked him.

Jessie and I drove back to Boston hauling a trailer with all her stuff. I cried many times on that trip. Jessie was tense but didn't want to talk about it. Her whole graduation had basically been sad and not a celebration. We stayed overnight in Pennsylvania and I had several drinks at a local restaurant and then I whipped out a cigarette and that shocked and angered her. As planned, we got back just two days before the Memorial Service. Ellen came in the next day.

Beverly and Rita had planned Jack's Memorial Service with just a little help from me. I decided to hold it at the Unitarian Church where we had been just before Jack and Ellen left for their skiing trip before his death. The minister asked if I was religious. I said I had been brought up as an Episcopalian but that I hadn't been to church for decades. No problem. Anything I wanted could be done. I said that if the minister wanted to say a few things that it was fine but I wanted no business about God. I asked Nancy, Ira and Jang-Ho to say something as well as Jack's brother and sister. I asked Jessie if she wanted to say something and suggested she read an essay she had written for college just that year about her father. I then asked Michael Lorimer, a friend, who was probably the best classical guitarist living, if he would play for the service. He came the day before and checked out the church and found the acoustics excellent.

The day of the service was perfect – a bright, sunny May day and in the low 70s. Beverly and Rita had arranged for the reception at Mass General on the lawn in front of the original hospital building. It was a short walk from the church. The buds and little leaves were on the trees. We got early to the church and a big screen had been set up at Nancy's direction. She said that I ought to see something before the service. She proceeded to play a video that had Jack talking briefly followed by Antonio Bocelli and Sarah Brightman singing "Time to Say Goodbye" while footage played of Jack in Venezuela with all the patients and team. Ellen and Jessie were also in it. The whole thing was completely heart-wrenchingly sad. Thank God I was able to see it before the service so I could stay composed when it played.

The church filled up with people. People came from the hospital and laboratory. Friends and family were there. Jack's patients came. Hundreds of neurologists from all over the country came. Michael blew them all away with his music. In between, there were some verses I had chosen. Everyone who spoke was incredibly articulate, sharing poignant moments but also managing to lighten the room with humor. Jessie and Jang-Ho were unbelievable in the way they captured the essence of Jack. Jessie said that Jack was her 'ground' in life and she loved him so much. Jack's father decided to speak at the last moment and was also wonderful. I finished up and was able to hold it together until the end when I broke down briefly in tears.

The whole thing had gone so well. It had all been incredibly moving and spiritual even though the word God had never been mentioned. Jack was well honored. I found it very comforting to see how many people came for both him and me. The reception went well also and then we went up to my apartment to sit out on the deck and listen to Michael's guitar.

The next day, I took the urn of ashes from the living room. Jack's dad, his wife, Jack's sister and brother and their spouses, Ellen and Jessie, Jang-Ho and his wife and Nancy Serrell came up to the graveyard in New Hampshire where Jack's mother was buried. Jack's dad had Jack's name and dates engraved on the opposite side of the gravestone. The graveyard was way off the road at the end of a field. The Strafford Graveyard. It had the graves of many long-term Bow Lake people dating back to the late 1700s. We all said our goodbyes and put notes in the urn and then the gravedigger covered it up. I planted a *Lamprocapnos spectabilis* ('bleeding heart') at the grave which blooms yearly.

20
· · · · ·

Recovery after Jack's Death

My life was quickly descending into a whirlpool of pain, self-loathing and despair. In the mornings, I couldn't get up. I had to set an alarm for the first time in my life. I hit the snooze button as often as possible while hiding under the covers and trying to catch up on my depressing dreams.

I spent a weekend at the lake, and while the weather and the water were beautiful to me everything was unhappy and hopeless. On these weekends, I started drinking in the late morning. By Sunday night, I had cleaned off a fifth of vodka and two bottles of wine. I also had no human contact the entire weekend. I told this to my therapist who said that if I wanted to meet new people that it was a bit absurd to escape to New Hampshire. The next weekend I stayed in Boston. It was clear and crisp and the fall colors were at their peak. But I had nothing to do. I called Jessie and she wasn't at her new apartment with friends across town, so I left a message. I talked to Nancy who said to call up an acquaintance from work. I called the acquaintance, but he wasn't home. I went out for a walk and people were all over the city – couples, families, dogs, bicycles, boats on the Charles River – but I was so alone and miserable. It was lonelier than in New Hampshire. I got a sandwich on the Common and came home. I fell asleep and when I woke up I spent the evening drinking and getting stoned.

The next day, Jessie called and we agreed to meet for a movie at 3:45 p.m. in Kendall Square. Three forty-five was a long way off though, so I took a nap and then started down to the movie theater shortly after 3 p.m. I couldn't find the theater. I found another theater and squatted on the sidewalk in front of it and waited until 4 p.m. I had no way to reach Jess. I walked and ran home. Jessie called after she got home and couldn't believe I had gone to the wrong place. She was exasperated. On the other hand, I just wanted to stick a knife in my heart (Figure 20.1). I tried Nancy but no answer. I finally left a message on her answering machine: "HELP!" Half an hour later, Jang-Ho called. "Hey, Anne. What are you doing tonight? We could come over with Leo. We'll bring the food." Leo was their baby. Rescue! Nancy had networked Boston to get someone on-site as soon as she could. She worked miracles for me. I can never thank her enough.

At work, I was tired, angry, sweaty and depressed, having to force myself to go from meeting to meeting and wishing I and

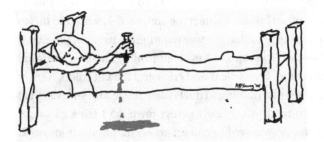

Figure 20.1 Sticking a knife in my belly.

everybody else were dead. I was always cold sober at work and at home when I was on call, but when I was not on call, I hit different liquor stores in sequence on my way home. There were many such stores directly on my way. If I went to a different one every night, it was unlikely that anyone would see me in the same store over and over and no one would assume I was a drunk. I'd pick up a fifth of vodka and a Lean Cuisine dinner to microwave and go home. Soon, I was relaxed and I'd start calling Ellen, Jessie or Nancy. On rare occasions, I called my mother. Ellen and Nancy were scared I might hurt myself and Jessie was understandably mad and fed up.

Some evenings, I'd drink less, and indeed in the summer of 2000, I stopped drinking for three weeks. I had no withdrawal symptoms, but by the time I hit three weeks, I was alert but just as depressed as well as irritable, explosive and angry. These feelings were as bad or worse than the feeling of hopeless depression. At least when I was drinking, I was taking out my anger and depression on myself more than others. Alcohol seemed the best thing.

In October, the American Neurological Association meeting was held in Boston. The meetings didn't start until later in the morning which meant I could sleep in. I went to all the functions and behaved myself except at the banquet, where I got pretty drunk. At midnight, I had a mile to walk home from Copley to Beacon Hill. I was staggering a bit and as I walked across the Public Garden the booze really hit me. Things were made worse by the fact that I had had a cigarette and I could feel that my blood pressure had gone way down. The hypotension and the alcohol combined made me stagger more and almost fall. That scared me. I felt lucky I wasn't mugged and hadn't fallen into a bush and passed out.

Later in the month, there was the Huntington Study Group (HSG) meeting in San Diego. By this time, I just couldn't care less. I drank all I could on the flight out and I had a small bottle of vodka with me in case the mini bar didn't exist. All through the

301

meeting, I drank from early afternoon on. People noticed and were worried. I didn't notice and I didn't care. Things just seemed beyond repair. I tried going through all the motions. I sat in the groups but couldn't offer any constructive comments or insights. The HD research was going fabulously. There was no need to be around. The sooner I was dead the better. One day I walked down to the beach in La Jolla with Jang-Ho. We saw rain showers off the coast and then a double rainbow. I recognized this view as a beautiful sight only with my rational brain, but I experienced none of the usual feelings of wonder and appreciation that nature can evoke. My limbic system was turned off. The pot of gold was filled with death and disaster.

This was also the year that my father had a bad fall and was found to have a ruptured Achilles tendon and two broken ribs. When I visited the farm that summer, he was thinner and not as lively or argumentative as he usually was. In September, back in Chicago, he was found to have metastatic bladder cancer and either metastases or other primary tumors.

That fall, my father got sicker and sicker. My mother called and said he had lost so much weight he was barely recognizable. He was sleeping 12 hours a day and was very weak when he was awake. She asked me to come out to visit but I didn't want to. I could barely take care of myself let alone anyone else, especially not my parents, with whom I still had a prickly relationship. I called up my dad's new internist and asked him to take a good look. The internist then admitted him to Lake Forest Hospital. Nothing particularly acute seemed to be going on but he was very weak and had lost almost 30 pounds. His chest x-ray showed a diffuse but not large new lesion and they recommended biopsy.

My mother was irate. "All you doctors want to do is make people uncomfortable and test them to death without any concern for their comfort," she said to me on the phone. "A biopsy! Through the nose! How brutal! He just can't go through all that!"

I tried to calm her down. I talked to my dad about it. His voice was weak but his resolve was strong. He was completely game to get the procedure. The bronchoscopy went well but unfortunately the biopsy was inconclusive. Now they wanted to do an open chest biopsy. I talked to both my parents and neither wanted something so invasive. I agreed. Dad was then transferred to the nursing facility at their retirement community. Now my mother had a new complaint. "Why are you doctors just giving up?"

I asked my mother to call her and Dad's old internist to see if he would come look at my dad. When I talked to the internist, he also indicated that my dad was very thin and weak. He'd detected a sixth nerve palsy, which I knew was often a sign of increased pressure in the brain, and a mild paralysis of the left side. I figured it was a metastasis to the right side of his brain that caused much of the weakness, double vision and trouble walking. I thanked my dad's old internist profusely and made reservations to go see my father on Saturday, November 4.

On Thursday night, I talked to Dad and he was mildly confused but still upbeat. I told him I'd see him soon.

The phone rang at 5:30 a.m., November 3, 2000. It was the nurse in Lake Forest. My father had died 30 minutes earlier in his sleep. I got on a 7:30 a.m. flight and was in Chicago by 9:30 a.m. My cousin, David, had gone to my mother's place to be with her. My mother shed a few tears but was otherwise very somber. David and I went to pick up my dad's things from his room at the nursing home. By the time my brother Peyton arrived late Friday afternoon, I was drunk. I had cleaned off some booze of my own as well as some of my mother's. I got through the rest of the weekend on my mother's booze.

After my dad died, I called my mother every day trying to pay her the attention she had denied me in the less than two years since Jack had died. Now we were both widows. At least my mother had had some warning that her husband was sick whereas I had suffered a sudden, visceral shock. Not to mention that Jack had been 51 years old, in the middle of his life while my father had lived to age 84 and had a happy, productive life. His death was not really upsetting to me. Three weeks after my father passed, we buried his ashes at the Buchwalter family plot in the cemetery after a brief ceremony.

A memorial service for my dad was scheduled for the Saturday after Thanksgiving. When I got there, I was informed that I was to say a few words at the service and, in fact, I was to be the first speaker. This was news to me but I wrote something up. Peyton and David also spoke. We all touched on similar traits of my father. Don't whine. Just do it. With inventiveness and pizzazz.

I spent the next weekend in New Hampshire, drunk and stoned, but I felt better once I spent a few hours outside and raked up all the leaves. On Wednesday of the next week, Sol Snyder came to Boston. We met that evening for dinner with the residents. I had two martinis and two glasses of wine. On Thursday, Sol gave the John B. Penney Jr. Memorial Lecture at Mass General and Nancy Wexler came to hear it (at the time I thought it was an odd thing for her to do). As expected, it was a great lecture. Nancy arranged to meet with Sol and me in my office after the lecture. By then, it was clear that something was up.

Sol sat down and Nancy pulled up a chair and said that I had to do something about my drinking and depression. They said I shouldn't have to feel this way. Grief is one thing, but I was over the edge and way too depressed for just grief. And the alcohol was making it worse. They both said they were worried and that I should go into the hospital. Whoa. I wasn't ready to hear this although I knew things were getting worse, not better. They wanted me to go right then and there. They mentioned Hazelden in Minnesota and Silver Hill in Connecticut. I said I would think about it, but they made me agree to go before letting me out of my office. Nancy called Joe Coyle, a psychiatrist at McLean

Hospital whom I'd known since medical school where he had had a laboratory next to Sol's. Nancy asked if he had any information on the two treatment centers. She stayed overnight in Boston and she and I arranged to see Joe Coyle the next day.

In the afternoon, I had to participate in a Harvard Medical School Forum on Medicine in the New Millennium that focused on neurodegenerative diseases. I chaired one session and gave a talk in another. At the reception afterward, Joe Martin announced the establishment at the Harvard Medical School of the John B. Penney, Jr. Professorship in Neurology for Parkinson's and Huntington's disease research at the Mass General.

Jack's family was there. Nancy was there. It was a wonderful event. What a mix of emotions I felt that day! I was ashamed that things had come this far! Wasn't I strong enough to cope with my grief on my own? But here was Joe Martin, the dean of the medical school, congratulating me on all I had done since Jack had died. Where was the truth? How could I be such a weak fuckup? Had I decided to go on with my life?

Friday, Nancy went with me to see Joe Coyle, who called the head of Silver Hill to arrange for me to be admitted on December 1 – the first day I was supposed to start attending on the inpatient service. I called up Alice Flaherty and asked if she was willing to be the only attending on the inpatient service for December. Normally, she and I shared the responsibility. She said yes. My other friends, Jang-Ho Cha and Diana Rosas, also said they would help if necessary.

I didn't tell my mother that I was going into an inpatient treatment facility. I feared the criticism or push from her to come and stay with her instead. If I had gone to stay with her, I can guarantee that I would have drunk myself to death. So the only people I told were Jack's family, Jessie and Ellen, Beverly, Alice, Jang-Ho, Walter Koroshetz and Zane.

The week before December 1, I had only three drinks and Nancy spent two nights with me. I had one appointment at McLean with a psychiatrist who specialized in people with alcohol and other psychiatric disorders including mood disorders, particularly women. I told her I was desperate for help and asked her if she would take me on as a patient when I got out of inpatient treatment. She said yes and I was relieved – she seemed like a good physician. She was young with a genuine smile. She asked questions rather than letting me flounder in long awkward silences.

I packed Thursday night. In the morning I finished several letters and stuff for work then headed to Silver Hill. The grounds were composed of residential-type houses on both sides of the road. The doctor's office building was quaint and looked reasonably comfortable in a classic New England way. Nancy met me there and was with me when I met the psychiatrist. I was assigned to K-House (Klingenstein House), but as soon as I had signed the admissions papers, I wasn't allowed to drive my car even the 100 feet to the parking lot. I did it anyway. My bags went with me to K-House. Psyche (it was really her name), the psych tech, checked me in and said she had to search all my bags and do a body search. No blades, knives, scissors, razors, books, computers, pills or papers. I had to strip for a body search. Every pocket and even the lining and hems of my coat were checked. I was going to be in a single room, thank God. Psyche checked my vitals (pulse, blood pressure and temperature) and I gave a urine sample. They loaded me up on Librium even though I knew I wasn't going to have alcohol withdrawal since I hadn't had withdrawal problems when I stopped drinking previously for more than three weeks. The psychiatrist at Silver Hill put me on medications for bipolar disorder, including a mood stabilizer.

I met the other people the next morning. K-House was coed and was the detox unit; it was a locked facility with frequent patient checks. There was a very gaunt man who had come in at

84 pounds and was now up to 100 pounds, an 18-year-old girl addicted to heroin, a couple of older women and an equal number of middle-aged men and women from various professions. People had different addictions – crack cocaine, alcohol, heroin and sedatives. One man hid his alcohol in his garden hose. Many people were admitted and discharged over the course of a week. Most commonly, people came in with their families after an intervention; they had been cornered by their families or friends and forced into treatment. Others came in after being arrested and the options were jail or rehab. Husbands had left wives and vice versa. DWIs (driving while intoxicated). Drug busts. Only a few came in on their own steam. Most people were pissed. Why can't I have my cell phone and my books? The food stinks. The staff are jerks. All very pissed off, very dependent people.

There were some commonalities, however. Most of us felt inadequate, unloved and desperate. Some people didn't give a shit about being alive or dead. Some just wanted to prove that they were really okay. Those were the dangerous ones, the ones that couldn't acknowledge that they had a problem. We spent our time going from one self-help group to another. We were watched like hawks. We had to line up and be counted as we left K-House to go to meals or make any other sojourns into the outdoor world. Every night there was a 12-step meeting. Alcohol, crack, opiates, gambling – everything on the 'anonymous' model. Everyone had the same basic problem – we pursued our addiction to the detriment of all other valuable lifetime activities. I certainly felt at home in this group and I loved the social interactions with the various 'inmates.' I started a K-House activist group to get access to exercise and swimming opportunities. I was told that 'exercise' was not advocated in the withdrawal phase. I agreed but felt that, after withdrawal, activity should be encouraged. We were given some very limited exercise time, but I started my own program of sit-ups, jumping jacks and leg lifts in my room.

I wasn't allowed to do any work. This was new and frustrating to me, but I soon learned that I needed my own time and that part of my problem was that everything in my life was Jack – including work. With Jack, of course, it was fun – a game. It was relaxing to talk about how the basal ganglia worked. Since his death, however, it wasn't fun and I hadn't learned how to fill the space otherwise.

I planned on staying at Silver Hill for three weeks and then going home to be with Jessie and Ellen. Gradually, I was able to tell my story without collapsing in tears. One Saturday, there was a family visiting session. Neither Jessie nor Ellen came to see me but Nancy did. I felt a little ray of hope. By getting better, perhaps I could renew my relationship with my daughters. I saw others who were getting better and people who had gotten through the program and were doing well. I felt very ambivalent, however; I wanted to be able to stop drinking but I didn't want to be like any of them. I had the distinct feeling that the program's objective was to wed everyone to the AA way of recovery, but I had problems identifying with the approach. One of the key AA tenets is to submit to a 'higher power' and I'm an agnostic and don't have any spiritual beliefs.

After two weeks, I graduated to an unlocked facility. I was also sent for a CT scan – which I had always been reluctant to have since that time in my twenties when I had been run over by the car and had fat emboli in my brain. Thank God I still had a brain. What's more, according to the CAT scan, it looked normal. On the day of my discharge, Nancy came to be with me and we learned the plan for the steps going forward. I would be in outpatient treatment at McLean Hospital until after the new year and then I would be followed twice a week by my new psychiatrist at McLean. Nancy and I hugged and kissed each other, and I thanked her profusely and she thanked *me*. I drove back to Boston to start a new life without alcohol and begin psychiatric therapy for my problems.

I quickly learned it wasn't a new life in most ways. I still went to work. I still had my lab. I still had my friends. And there was still no Jack. The apartment was still empty. Booze still called out to me every time I walked home and passed all those liquor stores. From treatment, I had learned that alcohol was cunning – drinkers personified alcohol as a friend, the only thing to offer comfort, or as a devil who could lead you astray. I kept this image in my mind. I wasn't going to answer the call of the bottle. I saw my new psychiatrist twice a week and she was superb. She diagnosed a lifelong history of untreated bipolar disorder. Finally, I had an explanation for the angry outbursts that had come over me for most of my life as well as the deep depressions I fell into at times – like when my patient in Michigan had committed suicide.

My psychiatrist quickly learned that I had trouble expressing my feelings. I couldn't put them into words. I had feelings but they didn't speak to me. They were nonverbal. Part of my work with her was learning how to articulate and express my feelings. And to recognize when my emotions were taking over.

Treatment had started me on a path but it was still a long and treacherous one. Many times I just didn't think I could go on and do this – learn to do without the need to artificially alter my mood. I hadn't done that in 32 years. I had no confidence that I had the personality I wanted without drugs. Could I enjoy anything? Could I relax at home and be comfortable with myself, reading a book, writing or watching a movie? These things were unknown to me because I hadn't done them in so long. Gradually, I learned to enjoy being sober with myself or others. Being sober also allowed me to develop my skills as a joke teller since now I could remember the punch lines.

Jack's death was still a great, raw wound that crippled me emotionally. I only wanted Jack to return and be with me. For the first two years after his death, I didn't even dream of him. I thought maybe it would help if I could at least feel his presence while I slept, but when he did come back to me in my dreams, I felt even worse. In the dreams, Jack was present even though we all acknowledged that he was dead. He never made love to me. He was always leaving or going out with other people. He said he didn't love me and I woke up deeply depressed (Figure 20.2). Thoughts of double-edged knives thrust and twisted between my ribs plagued my mind. I died with blood gushing from my chest. Then I began having dreams about Jack *every* night.

"No. You're dead," I said.

"No, I just organized my disappearance to Brazil. My family and I were the only ones to know. Dad helped me all along the way. Anne, I couldn't face you to say I no longer loved you. In fact, it's been years since I have felt an emotional bond with you. You are

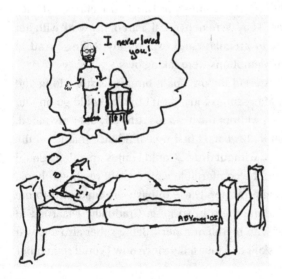

Figure 20.2 Jack coming back in my dreams to tell me he never loved me.

not attractive and you torture me with criticism. I can't live like this. You should be able to accept this three years after 'my death.'"

"But that's absurd. How could you 'pretend' to be dead? How could you lead me and others on? It has been unbearably painful and so many honored you. Now I find that you cared little about deceiving their friendship and nothing about your relationship with me."

"The facts are, unfortunately, that I don't love you and I have another girlfriend. I want a divorce. I'm going to fight you for every item I can. I also am going to fight for equal visiting rights with the girls."

"They are already of age and they can do what they want."

These nightly dreams continued for at least two years.

And then, they stopped. They weren't replaced by other dreams and I was no longer plagued by Jack telling me such terrible things. I had a few brief lapses in my struggle with alcohol, but each time I slipped, I came quickly back to sobriety. Each time, I lasted longer without drinking and I learned ways to stop the craving. Finally, I stopped for good and to this day I have no desire to drink. I learned how wonderful life is when you can wake up most mornings feeling well and not wanting to die. It had become such a routine feeling for me in my 32 years with intermittent severe depression. As part of my twice-weekly meetings with my psychiatrist, I learned that any return of the depressing Jack dreams meant I was falling into depression. But I could nip it in the bud with appropriate medication.

21
● ● ● ●

Building
the MassGeneral
Institute for
Neurodegenerative
Disease (MIND)

By 2001, two years after approval, the new building was designed, built and opened. The two main research floors were large and brightly lit by big windows. Faculty offices clustered near one end of the floor next to the common areas. There were no divisions between the labs. One set of benches flowed naturally into others. Four people worked at each bench. The benches stretched all around the outside of the floor, and in the middle there were internal rooms for core equipment like freezers, centrifuges, fancy microscopes and the like. There was an open stairway between the gathering areas on each floor where people could eat, get to know each other better or discuss life in general. One floor had a grand piano. Rudy Tanzi, an accomplished pianist, would often play in the breakout room. The whole design of MIND was to promote collaborations and the sharing of knowledge between investigators. Postdoctoral fellows, students, technicians and faculty mingled together daily and there was a current of excitement in the air.

About 30 independent faculty laboratory heads, so-called principal investigators (PI), occupied benches on the laboratory floors. Each PI had 5–15 people in their lab and in total about 300 people worked on the two main floors. The ground floor had conference rooms for lab meetings, seminars and meetings with donors or others. There were animal facilities to house transgenic animals and perform behavioral studies. Once the building opened, the laboratories filled up quickly. Right away, collaborations between labs developed and new grants to the National Institutes of Health were submitted and ultimately funded.

My lab and office moved to MIND and I dedicated two days a week to spend at the labs. Early on, I was still very depressed about Jack's death and I needed help to continue my research. Jack and I had done all our research together. Now, without him, I didn't have any enthusiasm or ambition. Without him, I couldn't keep up with the published papers. He had always read for me and my dyslexia now kept me uninformed. Zane and my previous trainees, Jang-Ho Cha and David Standaert, who both now had their own labs, helped me with my students, postdocs and technicians. They were incredibly close to me and did their best to make it possible for me to continue research in my lab. They wrote grants for me and closely followed all the spending we were doing on our grants. Without friends like them, I wouldn't have been able to keep my lab functioning. Fortunately, with their help, I was able to obtain funding for my lab through 2012.

MIND was successful in many ways. Not only were the PIs involved in cutting-edge research but side projects looking for new therapies were starting to show chemicals with some promise. Within five years, we were trying new potential drug therapies in animal models of Alzheimer's, Parkinson's, Huntington's diseases and ALS.

For HD research, we formed a team to devise new measures to assess several pathways thought to play a role in HD. Each pathway could be assessed by assays we designed in our labs. The assays were miniaturized and made into effective robotic high-throughput screens that could examine 'libraries' of thousands of potential drugs. We had six measures or assays, each examining a potential therapeutic step that could lead to a new therapy. Enough work in our labs on each step had already shown they had promise. We applied unsuccessfully to the National Institute for Neurological Disorders and Stroke for large grants to find new drugs for HD using these assays. We were very enthusiastic about our ideas, however, so despite the failed grants, we also negotiated with the pharmaceutical company Novartis to search for HD therapeutics. We negotiated a five-year project to pursue our ideas in collaboration with the company labs. This project taught me a lot about the difference in the way a drug company and academics approach a problem. Academics approach their hypothesis in an open-ended way whereas a company uses milestones and go/no-go decisions to reach their goals and minimize wasteful effort.

I was very active in all these efforts, traveling frequently to Washington, DC to defend our proposals at the National Institutes of Health. I also stayed close to Nancy, attending conferences with her and hanging out together. Now that the gene had been identified, we both thought therapies were right around the corner. Nancy's Hereditary Disease Foundation was making a major effort to find new ways of treating HD. HDF workshops were aimed at understanding each of the potential mechanisms of nerve cell death in the HD brain. I attended many of the workshops and I was also on the Scientific Advisory Board of the HDF that met yearly in Santa Monica, CA.

In those early years after Jack's death, I was elected president of the American Neurological Association – the second woman president. The association represented academic neurologists, and every member was elected to membership. I had served on a number of the association committees and my friends and colleagues nominated me for the position of president. This position required many meetings and public appearances. Following right afterwards, I was voted in as president of the 35,000-member Society for Neuroscience. As a perk of this position, I got to watch the Boston Red Sox win the Baseball World Series in 2004 for the first time in 86 years in the presidential suite of the San Diego Marriott. A lifelong Red Sox Fan, Jack would have loved to be there that day. During my time as president, I helped the Society build a new building in Washington, DC. These activities kept me busy and engaged. I'd come a long way since fighting on the elementary school playground – evidently I was liked and respected by my peers.

Ellen spent a year before medical school in New Zealand working on Huntington's disease in Sir Richard Faull's lab. I visited Ellen there and fell in love with the people and the country. Subsequently, I became chair of the Scientific Advisory Board of Sir Richard's Brain Research Centre in Auckland where I went every other year until 2019. Visiting with colleagues all over the world was such a perk of being in academic medicine and research.

In 2005, six years after Jack died, I received an email from my old eighth-grade and sometimes high school boyfriend, Stetson Ames. We were supposed to go to the senior prom together but his mother made him leave to spend the summer in Duxbury, Massachusetts before the prom and so I had no date. I hadn't seen or heard from him in over 35 years. He had joined the

Marines voluntarily in 1967 while all my other friends were trying to avoid the military. I knew that he had been in a terrible car accident on the military base that resulted in severe head and internal trauma. He gradually recovered and graduated from the University of Wisconsin. In the email, he said he was coming to Boston in May for his mother's memorial service in Duxbury at the Mayflower Cemetery. Would I like to go?

I didn't know what to say. I was about to leave on a trip to Chennai, India to give several lectures and didn't answer him until a month later. What should I say? What had he been up to? He wrote that he had retired from his job as a cop at the University of Wisconsin in Madison. His second wife had died. He had no children. I wrote back. "How many people have you killed? Do you have any tattoos? How about a girlfriend? Do you have one?"

"I haven't killed anyone. I have no tattoos and I don't have a girlfriend."

Seems promising. After six years of loneliness, perhaps it would be interesting to get together with Stets. He knew what it was like to lose a spouse. He wasn't intimidated by my position or accomplishments. He knew me as the scrappy kid he had had a crush on in high school and that was so nice. We emailed daily for the three months before the memorial service, and I invited him to come visit with me in Boston the week before the service. Beverly, Alice, Zane and Jang-Ho were all concerned because I hadn't seen him in so long and I just invited him to stay with me for a week. Nevertheless, he came to visit and I loved it. He was the same old guy I knew in high school. He was tall, lean, with a mustache and goatee. He still had a sneaky smile and a great sense of humor. He had given up all alcohol in the early 1980s and he didn't smoke. He was a Harley-Davidson motorcycle fanatic and rode all the time, preferably without a helmet. He was loving and very supportive of my work even though he was the opposite of Jack: a talkative, gun-loving, motorcycle-riding, fix-it man. Despite having no scientific training, Stets loved to attend neurology meetings with me as a guest. He had endless questions about how the nervous system worked. In smaller meetings, where again he was a guest and not a participant, he would raise his hand and ask a question and other people would whisper "he can't do that." One time at the American Academy of Neurology meetings, we were attending a session along with about 600 neurologists. Two famous neurologists on stage presented mystery neurology cases and asked questions for the audience. In one case, they presented a young man who was brought to the emergency room comatose and had a whitish foam around his mouth. They sent off a toxicology screen and it was negative for drugs. The people in the audience were guessing. "Maybe it's this or maybe it's that." But none were correct. Silence. Suddenly, Stets yelled out "Toluene!" (a potent solvent found in paint thinners and some types of glue). Toluene is so volatile that it's not readily picked up on toxicology screening. The neurologists asked Stets how he knew. Stets explained that, as a cop, he had found many kids getting high from sniffing glue and had seen similar symptoms.

In August 2005, he took me out to the Black Hills of South Dakota for the biggest annual rally of Harley-Davidson motorcycles in the world (Figure 21.1). Like me, Stets is irreverent. He drove around with no motorcycle helmet. He loved the speed, the wind through his hair and freedom. I rode as little as possible. We biked around the Black Hills. At the rally, I saw more motorcycles than I'd ever seen in my life. Three-quarters of a million motorcycles all zooming around the area at more than 80 decibels. It was crazy and the motorcycles and their owners were very diverse but festive. Hells Angels with tattoos all over, walking by the Blue Knights (law enforcement officers). People in leather vests or no shirt looking tough who I later found out were bankers, lawyers, doctors, neuroscientists, tattoo artists, construction workers – the whole

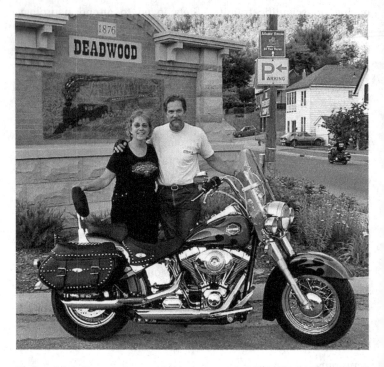

Figure 21.1 Stets and me with his motorcycle in the Black Hills of South Dakota.

group – were peaceful together. I wore blue jeans and a do-rag over my hair. Stets would comment that the bikes were "well dressed" when he saw a bike he liked. They had beautiful colors and decorations. It was quite an experience for me and despite my daughters' objections to ever riding a motorcycle, Stets and I got married a year later.

My mother was very pleased. Stets came from a prominent family and had gone to the same school as me. By that time, she was living in Palm Desert, California during the winters. When we visited her in

March, she said immediately to Stets, "Call me Louise, not Mrs. Young." It was the very opposite of what she had said to Jack.

As my mother neared 90, one time I found her in her bedroom lying on her bed, just staring at the ceiling. "What are you doing mom?" I said.

"I'm practicing to die in my sleep."

The next year, 2010, she did die. She left me $2 million in inheritance. I didn't really need the money, so after some thought, I donated $1 million to Mass General to set up a charitable annuity. I felt very positive about giving this donation because of the strength of the Mass General and its then fantastic leadership – Peter Slavin MD, Mass General president, and David Torchiana, president of the Mass General Physicians Organization. I arranged to have the money in my personal checking account. When I met with Slavin and Torchiana, I wrote the check for $1 million on my little checkbook and then signed it with great flourish. It was a win-win arrangement: I receive interest on the donation until I die and then the remainder goes to the hospital. This experience made me feel wonderful! I realized how rewarding it was to donate to a cause that would hopefully result in better understanding of and therapies for neurologic diseases. Fundraising became a future goal of mine.

Every year, we held two symposia at MIND on our successes in our search for new therapies for neurodegenerative diseases. Patients, family and friends were invited to hear from the MIND investigators about their discoveries. At the end of the presentations, participants could go on lab tours with the scientists. These activities were organized by Janice Hayes-Cha (Jang-Ho's wife who worked for me) and Krista McCabe from Development. Each year, these symposia lead to donations for MIND that could be used to support high-risk, high-payoff projects.

Nancy and I talked frequently at meetings and on the phone. I loved her. She had saved my life so many times – after Jack died, intervening to get me into treatment, and other times in Michigan when I was depressed or distraught. She had taught me so much about life. How to work hard for what you believe in and remain steadfast in times of crisis. How the differences between people have little to do with geographics or money or class but much to do with kindness, care and generosity.

As time went by, however, she seemed to be changing. Little things at first. Her writing became sloppier and sloppier. She stumbled from time to time and had occasional head movements. In the early years in Venezuela, Nancy used to ask me to do a neurological exam on her to check to make sure she had no signs of the disease. Then in the late 1990s, she stopped asking me. I didn't remind her. I couldn't face the thought of losing the other most important person in my life besides Jack. Nancy simply *couldn't* have HD. I worried and cried incessantly at the thought. Of course, I knew she was at risk but she was so smart – so well put together intellectually and physically. Jack had dropped dead instantly – too early but at least not after years of disability. If Nancy had HD, it would be a devastatingly long decline. I couldn't

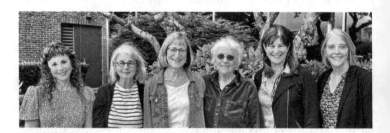

Figure 21.2 Women whose careers were all affected profoundly by Nancy's friendship and mentorship. Left to right: Sarah Tabrizi, Gill Bates, Diane Merry, me, Leslie Thompson and Beverly Davidson.

stand the thought. Several times, Nancy was at our apartment and I confronted her. "Do you think you have Huntington's?"

Every time, she reacted and gave it several minutes thought before replying, "No I really don't think I have it." She kept denying it.

Everybody who knew her came to me and said, "She has Huntington's, Anne. Why isn't she talking about it?"

And I'd say, "because she doesn't accept it." Nancy was in unbelievable denial and I was too. For at least four or five years I didn't want to see it. I made it go away.

Nevertheless, exciting research on HD and other neurodegenerative disorders was progressing and new pharmacological and genetic therapies were being developed in academic and industrial laboratories (Figure 21.2). Nancy and the HDF funded projects that examined the possibility of inserting small genes into the brains of animals to stop or slow the progression of the disease. I must say that I was skeptical of these approaches at first because I couldn't see how a gene could be delivered efficiently to the millions of human brain neurons. Overcoming the barriers, scientists like Beverly Davidson, then at the University of Iowa, were able to show in experimental animals that the technique worked. The idea was truly groundbreaking, and over the course of several years, companies began to adopt the approach and test it in humans.

22

• • • • •

Stepping Down after 21 Years

In 2012, at age 64, I decided to retire. I had been chief of service for 21 years. I felt strongly that leaders shouldn't stay too long in their positions. I didn't want to go past my prime. A new leader would bring a new financial package for the department, new recruits, new ideas and new expertise. The department was still at the cutting edge both clinically and in research, so I would be leaving a vibrant, productive faculty for the next leader. The hospital was also just finishing construction of a new clinical building. I had worked hard to get a commitment of three large floors for neurology/neurosurgery patients. It had a big modern ICU on one floor with a state-of-the-art MRI/PET scanner, the new machine to look at the brains of patients who could not be moved to get imaging on other floors. All the patient rooms were single occupancy and each had a window with a view of Boston.

Another reason for retiring was that my younger daughter, Ellen, had decided to become a neurologist. She had majored in neuroscience at Oberlin and then spent eight years completing an

MD/PhD program at Columbia University. Now she wanted to train in neurology at Mass General and was accepted into our program. I didn't want to be the chair if she was training at Mass General. It would have been nepotism if I continued. I had to step down. But now that Ellen was in the field, she and I could schmooze about neurology the way Jack and I once did.

Unlike many academics I knew, I didn't want to continue doing the same research I'd always done. Besides, without Jack, it was just no fun. By now, it was clear to me that I wasn't the one who would figure out the cause of HD or find an effective therapy. I had failed in this respect. At this point, it seemed reasonable to step aside and let others make those discoveries. Maybe I could keep my research going somehow, but why? If I were to try, it would be best to go on a year-long sabbatical to learn new techniques.

Many, many new techniques had been developed in the previous decade that made it possible to manipulate specific pathways and subsets of neurons in the brain. One amazing technique I was interested in was 'optogenetics.' This technique provided information that we could have only dreamed about back when we were examining the pathways of the basal ganglia. Optogenetics is the combination of light and genetics. Investigators can insert genes into specific types of nerve cells. The genes code for a light-sensitive protein hooked to an ion channel. When specific wavelength light is aimed at the cells, a channel opens to let in particular charged molecules like sodium, potassium or chloride. The result is that specific nerve cells' activity can be controlled with unique wavelengths of light. Channels sensitive to blue light increase the influx of sodium into the cell thereby exciting it. Yellow light activates channels allowing chloride into the cell thereby inhibiting it. Unlike our experiments in the 1980s, when we were unable to stimulate or inhibit pathways in alive, behaving animals, these new techniques have opened up a whole new vista of projects. In the

1980s, we had to kill the animal in order to determine the effects of a lesion. Now the animals can remain alive and their behaviors observed while different colored lights are flashed on the brain altering particular parts of the involved circuits. Optogenetics didn't give the animals Parkinson's but made the animal behave as if it did, at least temporarily.

I thought long and hard about what my path would be, discussing it frequently with my psychiatrist who I continue to see weekly. A sabbatical or no sabbatical?

If I retired, my lab space could go instead to a young investigator just starting a career. I had accumulated gift funds for my research program but now I could give them to those who could make good use of the funds to carry out experiments that could yield the preliminary data necessary for a new grant application. It made sense for the students of the people who'd invented optogenetics to see how much farther they could take these methods. They were the new generation just as I had once been. Such research had at least as much potential as *my* research to make important breakthroughs. Over the years, I had developed great pride in the people I had trained. They were smart, ambitious and hardworking. If I stepped aside, this would be another way to help them in their future endeavors.

The search committee for my replacement announced their choice – Merit Cudkowicz – a brilliant woman on our faculty who had established and directed our Program in Clinical Investigation. Her area of expertise is amyotrophic lateral sclerosis (ALS). She had also come down to Venezuela one year to work on the project. She was truly a person going from 'bench to bedside' by assessing potential new therapies discovered at the laboratory bench in humans using the best clinical trial designs. I was so happy that she was going to be the new chair of neurology. The second female chair in the history of the department. By the time she was recruited, several other female department chairs had been appointed at Mass General. Merit would be good for the department. Although she is not a basic scientist, she had the smarts to appoint excellent leaders of the department research laboratories.

In the end, I decided not to take a sabbatical. I arranged for all my postdocs and students to finish their projects and move on to new jobs, both at outside institutions and within Mass General. At 65, Zane retired shortly after I did. I moved my lab notebooks and papers to storage cages in MIND. As the prior chair of the department, I was given a new smaller office down the hall from the nice corner office I had occupied for years. Beverly also moved from her office to a cubicle near me.

To celebrate completing 21 years of service, I decided to organize a trip to the Galapagos. I had always wanted to go. I searched the internet and found an outfit with a boat that could accommodate 20 passengers. Why not invite 20 of my best friends to go on the trip? Not everybody could go, of course, but in the end the trip included Nancy, her sister Alice, David Housman and his wife, Gill Bates and her husband, Alice Flaherty and her family, my daughter Ellen and her boyfriend and others. The whole boat was occupied by good friends. Each day we landed on a different island and walked among the fearless birds, iguanas and tortoises. We snorkeled and swam with turtles and sea lions. Morning and afternoon activities gave us an appetite and the crew cooked up marvelous evening meals where we often discussed science and research on HD. It was an absolutely wonderful trip.

After stepping down, I continued to see patients but gradually began spending more and more time each week at our home in New Hampshire. I could work there. My patients had my cell phone number and could get in touch with me any time they wanted. I was in constant and frequent contact with Nancy; we were putting together grant applications and other projects. I became chair of the Scientific Advisory Board of Nancy's HDF, which entailed assigning grant reviewers, reviewing grants and running meetings. It gave me something of value to work on. I still felt useful to the field.

I started working with the development department at Mass General to fundraise for neurology. As chief of service, I had not inherited many funds to assist in the support of the department. When I began at Mass General, the department had only three endowed chairs. By the time I stepped down, we had ten. Having made my gift allowed me to feel comfortable asking others for donations. I worked with a team of young fundraisers at the hospital – Krista McCabe, Shawn Fitzgibbons and their colleagues. When a donor came forward, I discussed the person with their neurologist and then sent the person a letter inviting them for a visit with me and their neurologist. The purpose of the visit would be to discuss their neurologist's research work and see if the potential donor would be interested in supporting the research efforts. Any funds given would go to the investigator's personal 'sundry' account under their control. Most potential donors accepted the invitation. During the meeting, I could function as the interpreter, explaining in nonscientific language the meaning of the research findings. In this way I not only persuaded people to donate money but also stayed up to date on the science itself. We had great fun and great success over the ensuing years.

In 2014, one of our faculty, Nutan Sharma, began caring for a young man from the Philippines who had an illness called X-linked dystonia parkinsonism (XDP). This inherited disease started in midlife with twisting dystonic postures and shaking and symptoms similar to Parkinson's disease. It was only seen in those whose ancestry had lived on the island of Panay. Previous investigators had found the disease is caused by a gene on the X chromosome – one of our two sex chromosomes. XDP is one of the only dystonias accompanied by neurodegeneration of the striatum – the same brain area affected by HD. I was able to see videos of the affected people and I was struck by its similarity to aspects of HD. The family of Sharma's patient is very wealthy and asked if we could mount a research effort to find the gene and a cure for this disorder. They provided substantial funds to do just that.

I was appointed chair of the Scientific Advisory Board of the Collaborative Center for XDP (CCXDP). I was enthusiastic about joining the effort. We decided to take a similar approach as had been done for HD. I was able to go to the Philippines to see people affected by the illness. They were fishermen just like in Venezuela. They lived in abject poverty as in Venezuela and they too suffered a long, progressive and eventually fatal disease. The family that donated to start this project became very involved and organized the affected families in the Philippines to participate in research and tissue donation. Cris Bragg, a basic scientist in our department, took on the project's scientific leadership role in collaboration with the donors. In a few short years, the gene mutation was identified on the X chromosome. Work now goes on to find therapies. The project funded not only researchers at Mass General but also scientists at other institutions who had unique techniques and approaches.

My daughter, Ellen, joined the studies on XDP and has developed a brain bank for use by investigators around the world. Ellen specializes in movement disorders – in particular dystonia and HD. I'm proud that she continues at Mass General in the same field as her mom and dad, and I find it so rewarding to talk with her about the basal ganglia and how they work.

Stets and I spend much of our time in New Hampshire. There we have purchased the undeveloped lot next door and built a house with geothermal heating/cooling and solar panels. Jack's brother, Steve, and his boss hand-built the house. We have kept the old house, too, where the children and grandchildren stay. We have become involved in land conservation in our area, including conservation of the islands near us on the lake to ensure that they cannot be developed. The shoreline in our view was conserved by us also and we continue yearly support of local land conservation.

Over the years, I have tried to renew my relationship with Jessie and Ellen. I realized in retrospect how hard it was for them to lose their father and how I hadn't been able to help them as much as I wanted. Jessie got married several years after Jack died and spent time in the New York City Teaching Fellows program and worked in public schools before becoming a middle school science and math teacher at Friends Seminary (kindergarten through high school) in Manhattan, New York. She is now assistant head of the middle school. She is a joyful and enthusiastic teacher and she loves her job. In 2009, Eli, my first grandchild, was born. Because of her schedule as a teacher, Jessie and Eli have been able to spend every summer on the lake with us. Jessie and I like to cook. I usually make simple recipes but Jessie whips up all sorts of delicious concoctions. We alternate cooking the evening meals and holiday feasts. Having Jessie and Eli with us full time for two months a year has been a true gift. Jessie and Eli take hikes to explore nature and get exercise. Swimming and kayaking are also daily activities. In 2019, Alice Wexler and I took Jessie and Eli and one of his friends on a National Geographic cruise through the Alaska Inside Passage. We saw bubble-netting humpback whales, orcas, seals, mountain goats and glaciers. It was a magnificent trip.

Ellen has married as well and has an eight-year-old daughter, Amira, and a six-year-old son, Jack, born on my seventieth birthday. They come to New Hampshire often to swim, play, hike and be with their aunt Jessie and cousin Eli. Grandchildren have been such a joy. Sometimes when I am with them I think about what an attentive, interactive and playful grandfather Jack would have been. He had taken such good care of our daughters when they were growing up and had wonderful parenting skills.

Beverly retired in 2015, and I stopped seeing patients when she left. She and I had always taken care of my patients as a team. She knew my patients well and could always find me if a problem arose. I valued her input on each person. Seeing patients without her would be difficult and I wasn't motivated to set up a new appointment system. I didn't renew my medical license.

23

• • • • •

Hope for the Future of Disorderly Movements

In many ways, things in medicine have improved since I began my career. Many neurological illnesses such as Parkinson's disease, epilepsy, multiple sclerosis, myasthenia gravis and others now have vastly improved therapies. At the same time, doctors face challenges, particularly in the time wasted on paperwork and extensive documentation required by insurance companies that leave less time for actual patient interactions. Although women have made up at least 50 percent of medical student classes for years now, their promotion to the highest academic and leadership levels is still a challenge. One exception is Anne Klibanski, MD, an accomplished neuroendocrinologist from the Mass General who is now the CEO of the Mass General Brigham (a result of the merger) – the largest research-based hospital system in the US.

Mental health issues are less stigmatized and more understood than in my youth. I could have benefited from help earlier in life. Treatments for mental disorders have improved dramatically also.

I was fortunate to have Jack who kept me safe all those years we were together. After his death, working with a therapist made it possible for me to make order out of the disorder. The hardest part was taking that necessary first step.

We've come so far since my early studies in Sol's lab. We know there are not just four but dozens of neurotransmitters – often several in a single neuron. Furthermore, there are many different subtypes of neurotransmitter receptors and drugs have been targeted to each one of them. New technologies such as optogenetics allow the manipulation of the basal ganglia circuits in living animals. A parallel approach called chemogenetics may soon become available for humans. As predicted by Jack, Roger and me back in 1989, deep brain stimulation is used routinely to treat Parkinson's disease and tremors. Focused ultrasound methods of lesioning deep brain structures can now be done for these disorders without any brain surgery.

Since the human genome was sequenced in 2000, aided to a large extent by the work on HD, it is now easy to identify the mutations for most diseases – the challenge is to develop treatments to help them. Small pieces of genetic material have been designed to turn down the HD gene or its modifiers. These approaches are being investigated in clinical trials and already several show promise. Small molecules are being developed for HD therapy and hopefully they will prove effective as a simple oral treatment. Despite the challenges, there are many reasons why effective treatments for disorderly movements and neurodegenerative disorders will be developed in the next decade. Ideally, the therapies will be applied around the world, including developing countries.

Despite my greatest fears, by 2015, it was becoming impossible for me to deny Nancy's signs of HD. My best friend was being taken away by the same illness that we had devoted our careers to studying. She lost a great deal of weight and her walking was unsteady. I talked again with her but she still said she thought she didn't have the disease. It was ripping me apart. Because she denied it, she closed the door to talking about it. I wanted so much to help her. I talked tangentially about the issue but she was so smart she could see through my motives. Nancy's sister, Alice, became a close friend as she tried to navigate the situation too. We both hoped Nancy would join a clinical trial. Several promising therapies were being tested. Eventually Nancy agreed, but to be eligible to join the trial there was only one catch: She had to get a formal diagnosis. Upon asking, her neurologist gave her a clinical diagnosis of symptomatic Huntington's disease. Despite suspecting it, the diagnosis was a huge blow to Nancy. It was also a knife through my heart since I couldn't continue to deny what was happening. She had spent her whole life trying to cure this disease and now she had it. To top it off, she was too old for the most promising trial, antisense oligonucleotides (ASOs), run by Sarah Tabrizi and her trainee Ed Wild at University College London in collaboration with Roche Pharmaceuticals. By the time Nancy was given an exception to the inclusion rules, the trial was suddenly stopped as the treatment was making people *worse*.

Despite this heart-rending disappointment, I am optimistic about the future. New effective therapies for HD and other neurodegenerative diseases are in clinical trials. Sarah, Ed and their collaborators are trying to figure out why the ASO trial failed. New trials of ASOs are underway – several under Sarah's direction. Another recent early phase trial in the treatment of HD has just been shown to have positive results. Multiple approaches are being investigated in clinical trials and already several show promise. Small molecules are being developed for HD therapy and hopefully they will prove effective as a simple oral treatment. Parkinson's and ALS therapies are also in the pipeline. In Alzheimer's disease, an antibody that clears amyloid is available for clinical treatment of early Alzheimer's disease.

I recently Zoomed with Nancy, who now lives in a lovely New York City apartment on Riverside Drive with wonderful views of the Hudson River and 24/7 aides who attend to her needs. Over our Zoom call, Nancy was excited that her Hereditary Disease Foundation was going to fund three large and extremely innovative research grants that promise the application of novel approaches to find HD therapies. Despite her physical impairment, Nancy remains intellectually very engaged. Our weekly Zoom calls include her sister, Alice, and sometimes other friends and scientists. Although we often share racy jokes and stories and reminiscences of our adventures in Venezuela and Peru, Nancy likes to bring us back to discussions of the new research projects. Over Zoom, I feel I can at least communicate with her regularly. I occasionally visit her in New York to be with her personally. She was my savior so many times but I have not been able to save her. Nevertheless, Nancy has shown the world it is possible to live a rich life, make unparalleled discoveries, help thousands with genetic disease and support the careers of so many young scientists, especially women, all while living *with* Huntington's disease. Working with her all these years, I have learned so much about disorderly movements and disorderly thinking. Hopefully, these illnesses will become things of the past in the next generation.

Acknowledgments

I have been working on this manuscript since Jack died. When two good friends named Alice – Alice Wexler and Alice Flaherty – encouraged me to turn it into a book that could be of interest to young scientists and women, I decided to give it a try. Alice Flaherty hooked me up with writer Karen Propp and we began working together to shape and develop first a proposal and then a manuscript. Karen has been a wonderful editor and collaborator, and the book couldn't have been completed without her. The two of us were joined by Hannah Applebaum as our assistant. She has been a valuable member of my helpers, and I am so very grateful to both of them. Anna Whiting at Cambridge University Press was a thoughtful guide throughout the process and her senior editorial assistant, Camille Lee-Own, provided important input as well.

My career would not have been possible without my many mentors starting with Herb Philipsborn, my pediatrician; Anne Gounaris, my Vassar research supervisor; Sol Snyder, my graduate school mentor; Sid Gilman, my chair at the University of Michigan; Nancy Wexler and her partner Herb Pardes. Gerald Austen, Sam Thier, Jim Mongan, Peter Slavin and David Torchiana were steadfast supporters throughout my time at Mass General.

Zane Hollingsworth worked with me for 35 years and helped everything I did succeed. His measured, thoughtful, fair recommendations always made sense and people trusted him. With him, my lab functioned efficiently and our department faculty had confidence that he would support their needs as well.

Beverly Mahfuz was a partner with me in running the neurology department at Mass General for two decades. With her constant help, she made my accomplishments possible. She read all my letters and emails to the end and flagged all items that needed attention. She rapidly learned my style, strengths and weaknesses. She taught the students, residents and junior faculty how to interact with me.

My psychiatrist, Shelly Greenfield, and I have discussed all aspects of the book together and she helped me define the most important parts. She has also kept me well over the last 24 years.

I have mentioned a few of my trainees in the manuscript but there are many others who worked in the lab with me and Jack. All of you were part of our scientific family. You all added to the joy in my life. I haven't forgotten you.

Many people read the manuscript as a work-in-progress and offered valuable feedback which shaped it for the better. I am grateful for time and insights given by: Jang-Ho Cha and Janice Hayes-Cha, Janet and Paul Cronin, Rebecca Eaton, Alice Flaherty, John Herman, Anne Jardim, Beverly Mahfuz, Krista McCabe, Brit Nicholson, Steve Penney, Susan MacAlden, Ann Sarowsky, Patti and David Taylor and Alice Wexler.

My daughters have been very supportive of me in this effort although certain chapters are painful for them. They have made important suggestions that I have incorporated. Stets has also been a constant backer throughout my endeavors and contributed adventures of his own. He encouraged my goal of having three hours a day of uninterrupted work time.

Finally, I want to thank all my patients over the years. I tried my best to help all of you. In particular, I want to thank the wonderful HD families in Venezuela, Peru and Spain who made finding the HD gene mutation possible.

Index

Index

Index

338

Movement Disorders, 196
Movement Disorders Clinic, 140
Mrs. Moore, 29
myopathy, 117
Mystic River, 296

naloxone, 91
nanny (full-time, live-in), 124
National Geographic, 122
National Institute of Neurological
    Disorders and Stroke (NINDS),
    136, 253, 314
National Institutes of Health (NIH), 57
    grant application, 129, 135, 151, 313
    Office of Scientific Integrity, 283
    traveling to defend proposals, 314
Natural History, 122
Negrette, Americo, 158
neuroblastoma, 128
neurodegenerative disorders, near-
    future effective treatments for, 331
neurogenetics, 255
neurological evaluation, 260
neurology, 81, 122
    board certification examination in,
    144
    pediatric neurology, 123, 125
    residency in, 106–134
    what it involves, 247
Neurology, 122
neurology 'grand rounds,' 7
Neurology Match, 266
neuromuscular disease, 255
neuropathology, Jack's fellowship in at
    the Veterans Health
    Administration Hospital, 129
neuropsychiatric disorders, first
    exposure to, 28
neurosurgery, introduction to while in
    medical school, 74
neurotoxins, 95
neurotransmitter receptors
    measuring, 149
    measuring autoradiographically, 173
    types and subtypes of, 331

neurotransmitters, 59, 331
    basal ganglia and, 172–192
    homocarnosine investigation, 84, 89
neurovirology, 130
New England Journal of Medicine, 122
New England Nuclear Corporation, 96
New England Organ Bank, 4, 7
New Hampshire lake house, 262
New York City Teaching Fellows
    program, 328
New York Times
    HD gene discovery, 259
    marker discovery, 208
Newman, Sarah, 130
Night Watch, 9
NIH. *See* National Institutes of Health
NINDS (National Institute of
    Neurological Disorders and
    Stroke), 136, 253, 314
NMDA receptors, 267
Nobel Prize in Physiology or Medicine
    for 1970, 59
nongovernmental foundation grants,
    136
norepinephrine, 59
Northwest Flight 255 crash on take-off,
    197
NOVA crew, 210, 212, 221
Novartis, 314

O'Grady, Sherri, 250, 256, 294
'observers on the scene,' 110, 121
OKN (optokinetic nystagmus) tape, 164
Olson, Jim, 147
Olympic Peninsula, 104
opiate antagonist, 91
opiate overdose, 91
opiate receptor, 91, 98
optogenetics, 323, 331
optokinetic nystagmus (OKN) tape,
    164
organ donations, 4, 8
Orrick, Pigeon, 33
Oster-Granite, Mary Lou, 101, 102
our honeymoon, 81

Printed in the United States
by Baker & Taylor Publisher Services